影像解剖学系列图谱

总主编 刘树伟 林祥涛

Atlas of Imaging Anatomy: **Abdomen**

腹部影像
解剖图谱

主 编 汤煜春 娄 丽

山东科学技术出版社

图书在版编目（CIP）数据

腹部影像解剖图谱 / 汤煜春，娄丽主编 . —济南：山东科学技术出版社，2020.1

（影像解剖学系列图谱 / 刘树伟，林祥涛总主编）

ISBN 978-7-5331-8235-9

Ⅰ . ①腹… Ⅱ . ①汤… ②娄… Ⅲ . ①腹腔疾病－影象诊断－人体解剖学－图谱 Ⅳ . ① R572.04-64

中国版本图书馆 CIP 数据核字（2018）第 141977 号

腹部影像解剖图谱
FUBU YINGXIANG JIEPOU TUPU

责任编辑：徐日强

装帧设计：孙　佳

主管单位：山东出版传媒股份有限公司

出　版　者：山东科学技术出版社

地址：济南市市中区英雄山路 189 号

邮编：250002　电话：（0531）82098088

网址：www.lkj.com.cn

电子邮件：sdkj@sdcbcm.com

发　行　者：山东科学技术出版社

地址：济南市市中区英雄山路 189 号

邮编：250002　电话：（0531）82098071

印　刷　者：山东彩峰印刷股份有限公司

地址：潍坊市福寿西街 99 号

邮编：261031　电话：（0536）8216157

规格：32 开（125mm×190mm）

印张：5　字数：100 千　印数：1~3000

版次：2020 年 1 月第 1 版　　2020 年 1 月第 1 次印刷

定价：20.00 元

总主编 刘树伟 林祥涛

主　编 汤煜春 娄　丽

编　者（以姓名笔画为序）

　　　　王小洪（山东大学齐鲁医学院）

　　　　汤煜春（山东大学齐鲁医学院）

　　　　肖　敏（山东大学齐鲁医学院）

　　　　娄　丽（山东省千佛山医院）

　　　　盖新亭（山东大学齐鲁医学院）

总　前　言

超声、CT 和 MRI 等现代断层影像技术发展迅速，已成为当今临床诊治疾病的必备工具。不仅影像科医师要正确地阅读超声、CT 和 MR 图像，而且临床各科医师均要娴熟地应用断层影像技术诊治疾病。影像解剖学是正确识别疾病超声、CT 和 MR 图像的基础，是介入及手术治疗疾病的向导。因此，只有掌握了影像解剖学，才能准确判读和应用超声、CT 和 MR 图像。1993 年以来，在中国解剖学会断层影像解剖学分会领导下，山东大学齐鲁医学院断层影像解剖学研究中心共举办了 25 届全国断层影像解剖学及其临床应用学习班，报名参加者络绎不绝。这充分说明了断层影像解剖学的重要性，我们也深深感到自己责任的重大。在长期的教学过程中，教师和学员均感到编写一套以活体超声、CT 和 MR 图像为基础的"影像解剖学系列图谱"的重要性和必要性。为此，我们组织山东大学从事断层影像解剖学研究和教学的有关人员，编写了这套"影像解剖学系列图谱"，以期能满足临床各科医师学习正常超声、CT 和 MR 图像的需求。

为适应不同临床学科医师学习影像解剖学的专业需求，本套"影像解剖学系列图谱"分成了 6 个分册，包括《颅

1

脑影像解剖图谱》《头颈部影像解剖图谱》《胸部影像解剖图谱》《腹部影像解剖图谱》《盆部与会阴影像解剖图谱》和《脊柱与四肢影像解剖图谱》。在编写过程中，根据临床实际要求和方便读者阅读的原则，本套图谱追求以下特色：（1）系统性，从临床应用角度，全面系统地介绍人体各部位的正常超声、CT 和 MR 图像；（2）连续性，以健康中青年志愿者连续断层图像介绍人体各部的连续横断层、矢状断层和冠状断层解剖；（3）先进性，利用当今临床上最新的设备制作超声、CT 和 MR 图像，并吸纳了国内外断层影像解剖学的最新研究成果；（4）实用性，以解剖部位划分分册，版本采用小开本以方便读者随身携带，在图像选择和结构标注上以临床常用者为主；（5）可扩展性，每部分册末均附有一定数量的推荐读物，供欲进一步详细阅读者参考，使本套图谱具有一定的扩展性。

本套图谱的解剖学名词主要参照全国科学技术名词审定委员会公布的《人体解剖学名词（第二版）》（科学出版社 2014 年出版）。当《人体解剖学名词（第二版）》与临床习惯叫法不同时，则采用临床常用者。

本套图谱主要以临床各学科医师为主要读者对象，亦可供解剖学教师、临床医学和基础医学各专业硕士与博士研究生参考。

由于作者水平所限，书中疏漏甚至错误之处在所难免。恳请读者不吝赐教，以便再版时更正。

刘树伟　林祥涛
2019 年 11 月于济南

前　言

《腹部影像解剖图谱》主要以图谱形式展示具有重要临床意义的解剖学结构，力求简明实用、小巧灵便、便于随身携带及随时随地查阅。全书包括7章，共有图片146幅，分别为：腹部CT横断层图像20幅，腹部CT矢状断层图像27幅，腹部CT冠状断层图像19幅，腹部MR横断层图像20幅，腹部MR矢状断层图像25幅，腹部MR冠状断层图像20幅和腹部B超图像15幅。

影像图片主要由山东省医学影像学研究所和山东省立医院影像科提供。MR图像由3.0T SIEMENS磁共振扫描仪采集，序列为T_2加权图像；CT图像由SIEMENS CT扫描仪采集，并经MPR重建获得；B超图像由TOSHIBA Aplio500和GE LOGIQ 9彩色多普勒超声扫描仪采集，探头频率为3.5~5.0 MHz。

本图谱是人体解剖学和医学影像学工作者的联袂之作，可供影像学医师、普外科医师、泌尿外科医师、妇产科医师、解剖学教师和医学院校学生学习使用。

腹部脏器多，结构复杂，且变异较多。尽管作者做了最大努力，但书中仍可能出现不少错误和不妥之处，恳请广大读者谅解并不吝赐正，以便再次修订时参考。

汤煜春　娄　丽

2019 年 11 月

目　录

第一章 腹部横断层 CT 图像

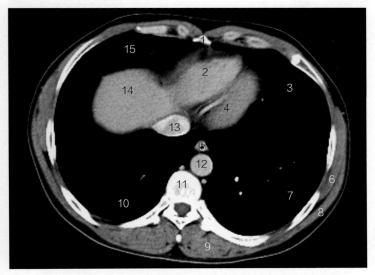

图 1-1 经膈右穹隆的横断层 CT 图像

1　胸骨体 body of sternum

2　右心房 right atrium

3　左肺上叶 superior lobe of left lung

4　左心室 left ventricle

5　食管 esophagus

6　前锯肌 serratus anterior

7　左肺下叶 inferior lobe of left lung

8　背阔肌 latissimus dorsi

9　竖脊肌 erector spinae

10　右肺下叶 inferior lobe of right lung

11　第 9 胸椎椎体 body of 9th thoracic vertebrae

12　胸主动脉 thoracic aorta

13　下腔静脉 inferior vena cava

14　肝右叶 right lobe of liver

15　右肺中叶 middle lobe of right lung

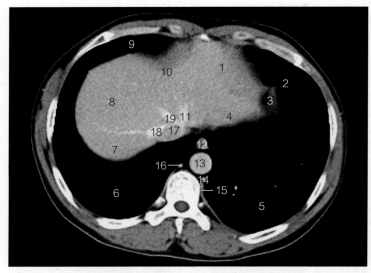

图 1-2　经第二肝门的横断层 CT 图像

1　心脏 heart	2　左肺上叶 superior lobe of left lung
3　胃底 fundus of stomach	4　肝左外叶 left lateral lobe of liver
5　左肺下叶 inferior lobe of left lung	
6　右肺下叶 inferior lobe of right lung	
7　肝右后叶 right posterior lobe of liver	
8　肝右前叶 right anterior lobe of liver	
9　右肺中叶 middle lobe of right lung	
10　肝左内叶 left medial lobe of liver	11　肝左静脉 left hepatic vein
12　食管 esophagus	13　胸主动脉 thoracic aorta
14　半奇静脉 hemiazygos vein	15　左膈脚 left crus of diaphragm
16　奇静脉 azygos vein	17　下腔静脉 inferior vena cava
18　肝右静脉 right hepatic vein	19　肝中静脉 middle hepatic vein

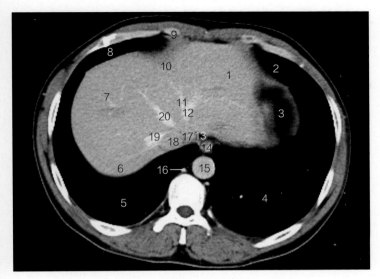

图 1-3　经食管裂孔的横断层 CT 图像

1　肝左外叶 left lateral lobe of liver	2　左肺上叶 superior lobe of left lung
3　胃底 fundus of stomach	4　左肺下叶 inferior lobe of left lung
5　右肺下叶 inferior lobe of right lung	
6　肝右后叶 right posterior lobe of liver	
7　肝右前叶 right anterior lobe of liver	
8　右肺中叶 middle lobe of right lung	
9　肝镰状韧带 falciform ligament of liver	
10　肝左内叶 left medial lobe of liver	11　左叶间静脉 left interlobar vein
12　肝左静脉 left hepatic vein	
13　静脉韧带裂 fissure for ligamentum venosum	
14　食管 esophagus	15　胸主动脉 thoracic aorta
16　奇静脉 azygos vein	17　肝尾状叶 caudate lobe of liver
18　下腔静脉 inferior vena cava	19　肝右静脉 right hepatic vein
20　肝中静脉 middle hepatic vein	

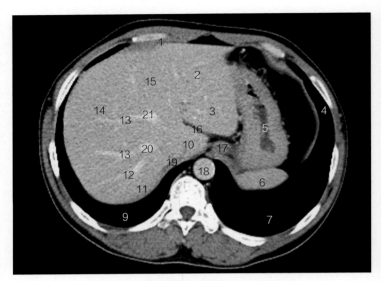

图 1-4　经食管腹段的横断层 CT 图像

1　肝镰状韧带 falciform ligament of liver

2　肝左静脉 left hepatic vein　　　3　肝左外叶 left lateral lobe of liver

4　左肺上叶 superior lobe of left lung　　　5　胃体 body of stomach

6　脾 spleen　　　7　左肺下叶 inferior lobe of left lung

8　半奇静脉 hemiazygos vein

9　右肺下叶 inferior lobe of right lung　　　10　肝尾状叶 caudate lobe of liver

11　肝右后叶 right posterior lobe of liver

12　肝门静脉右后上支 right posterosuperior branch of hepatic portal vein

13　肝门静脉右前上支 right anterosuperior branch of hepatic portal vein

14　肝右前叶 right anterior lobe of liver　　　15　肝左内叶 left medial lobe of liver

16　静脉韧带裂 fissure for ligamentum venosum

17　食管腹段 abdominal part of esophagus

18　胸主动脉 thoracic aorta　　　19　下腔静脉 inferior vena cava

20　肝右静脉 right hepatic vein　　　21　肝中静脉 middle hepatic vein

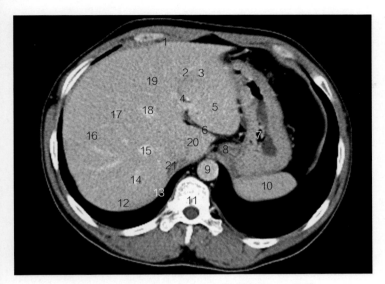

图 1-5 经肝门静脉左支角部的横断层 CT 图像

1　肝镰状韧带 falciform ligament of liver

2　肝门静脉左外上支 laterosuperior branch of left hepatic portal vein

3　肝左静脉 left hepatic vein

4　肝门静脉左支角部 angular part of left hepatic portal vein

5　肝左外叶 left lateral lobe of liver

6　静脉韧带裂 fissure for ligamentum venosum

7　胃体 body of stomach　　　　　　　8　胃贲门部 cardiac part of stomach

9　胸主动脉 thoracic aorta　　　　　　10　脾 spleen

11　第 11 胸椎椎体 body of 11th thoracic vertebrae

12　肝右后叶 right posterior lobe of liver　13　肝裸区 bare area of liver

14　肝门静脉右后上支 right posterosuperior branch of hepatic portal vein

15　肝右静脉 right hepatic vein

16　肝右前叶 right anterior lobe of liver

17　肝门静脉右前上支 right anterosuperior branch of hepatic portal vein

18　肝中静脉 middle hepatic vein　　　19　肝左内叶 left medial lobe of liver

20　肝尾状叶 caudate lobe of liver　　　21　下腔静脉 inferior vena cava

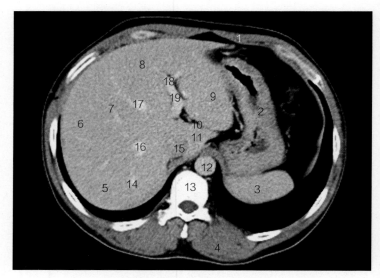

图 1-6　经肝门静脉左支矢状部的横断层 CT 图像

1　腹直肌 rectus abdominis　　2　胃体 body of stomach

3　脾 spleen　　4　竖脊肌 erector spinae

5　肝右后叶 right posterior lobe of liver

6　肝右前叶 right anterior lobe of liver

7　肝门静脉右前上支 right anterosuperior branch of hepatic portal vein

8　肝左内叶 left medial lobe of liver　　9　肝左外叶 left lateral lobe of liver

10　静脉韧带裂 fissure for ligamentum venosum

11　肝尾状叶 caudate lobe of liver　　12　胸主动脉 thoracic aorta

13　第 12 胸椎椎体 body of 12th thoracic vertebrae

14　肝门静脉右后上支 right posterosuperior branch of hepatic portal vein

15　下腔静脉 inferior vena cava　　16　肝右静脉 right hepatic vein

17　肝中静脉 middle hepatic vein

18　肝门静脉左支囊部 sac part of left hepatic portal vein

19　肝门静脉左支矢状部 sagittal part of left hepatic portal vein

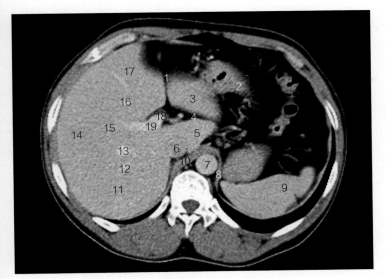

图 1-7　经肝门的横断层 CT 图像

1　肝圆韧带裂 fissure for ligamentum teres hepatis

2　胃体 body of stomach   3　肝左外叶 left lateral lobe of liver

4　肝胃韧带 hepatogastric ligament   5　肝尾状叶 caudate lobe of liver

6　下腔静脉 inferior vena cava   7　胸主动脉 thoracic aorta

8　左膈脚 left crus of diaphragm   9　脾 spleen

10　右膈脚 right crus of diaphragm

11　肝右后叶 right posterior lobe of liver

12　肝门静脉右后上支 right posterosuperior branch of hepatic portal vein

13　肝右静脉 right hepatic vein

14　肝右前叶 right anterior lobe of liver

15　肝门静脉右前上支 right anterosuperior branch of hepatic portal vein

16　肝中静脉 middle hepatic vein   17　肝左内叶 left medial lobe of liver

18　肝门静脉左支横部 transverse part of left hepatic portal vein

19　肝门静脉右支 right hepatic portal vein

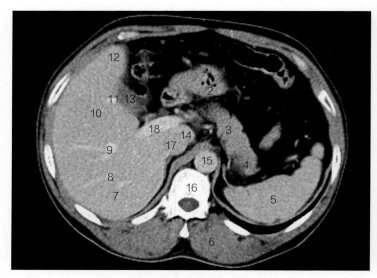

图 1-8　经肝门下方的横断层 CT 图像

1	腹直肌 rectus abdominis	2	胃体 body of stomach
3	胰体 body of pancreas	4	胰尾 tail of pancreas
5	脾 spleen	6	竖脊肌 erector spinae
7	肝右后叶 right posterior lobe of liver	8	肝右静脉 right hepatic vein

9　肝门静脉右后下支 right posteroinferior branch of hepatic portal vein

10	肝右前叶 right anterior lobe of liver	11	肝中静脉 middle hepatic vein
12	肝左内叶 left medial lobe of liver	13	胆囊底 fundus of gallbladder
14	肝尾状叶 caudate lobe of liver	15	胸主动脉 thoracic aorta

16　第 12 胸椎椎体 body of 12th thoracic vertebrae

17　下腔静脉 inferior vena cava

18　肝门静脉右支 right hepatic portal vein

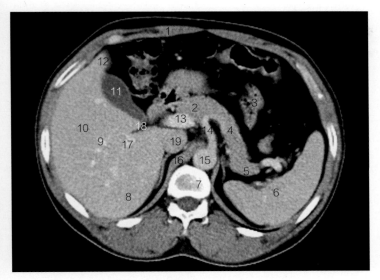

图 1-9　经腹腔干的横断层 CT 图像

1　腹直肌 rectus abdominis　　　　　2　胰颈 neck of pancreas

3　胃体 body of stomach　　　　　　4　胰体 body of pancreas

5　胰尾 tail of pancreas　　　　　　6　脾 spleen

7　第 12 胸椎间盘 12th thoracic intervertebral disc

8　肝右后叶 right posterior lobe of liver

9　肝右静脉前根 anterior root of right hepatic vein

10　肝右前叶 right anterior lobe of liver　　11　胆囊体 body of gallbladder

12　肝左内叶 left medial lobe of liver　　13　肝门静脉 hepatic portal vein

14　腹腔干 celiac trunk　　　　　　15　腹主动脉 abdominal aorta

16　右膈脚 right crus of diaphragm

17　肝门静脉右后下支 right posteroinferior branch of hepatic portal vein

18　肝门右切迹 right notch of portal hepatis

19　下腔静脉 inferior vena cava

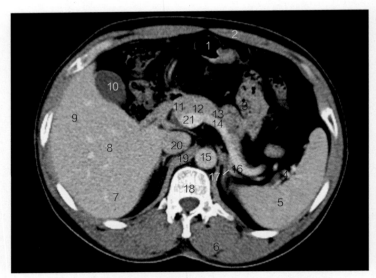

图 1-10　经肝门静脉合成处的横断层 CT 图像

1	横结肠 transverse colon	2	腹直肌 rectus abdominis
3	胃体 body of stomach	4	脾门 hilum of spleen
5	脾 spleen	6	竖脊肌 erector spinae

7 肝右后叶 right posterior lobe of liver

8 肝门静脉右后下支 right posteroinferior branch of hepatic portal vein

9	肝右前叶 right anterior lobe of liver	10	胆囊体 body of gallbladder
11	胰头 head of pancreas	12	胰颈 neck of pancreas
13	胰体 body of pancreas	14	脾静脉 splenic vein
15	腹主动脉 abdominal aorta	16	左肾上腺 left suprarenal gland

17 左膈脚 left crus of diaphragm

18 第 1 腰椎椎体 body of 1st lumbar vertebrae

19	右膈脚 right crus of diaphragm	20	下腔静脉 inferior vena cava

21 肠系膜上静脉 superior mesenteric vein

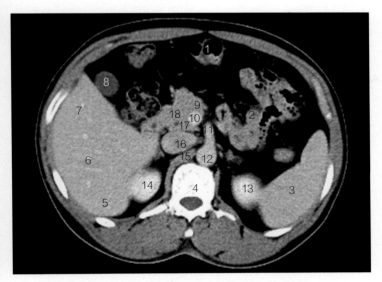

图 1-11　经肠系膜上动脉的横断层 CT 图像

1　横结肠 transverse colon　　　　2　胃 stomach

3　脾 spleen

4　第 1 腰椎椎体 body of 1st lumbar vertebrae

5　肝右后叶 right posterior lobe of liver

6　肝右静脉前根 anterior root of right hepatic vein

7　肝右前叶 right anterior lobe of liver　　8　胆囊 gallbladder

9　胰颈 neck of pancreas

10　肠系膜上静脉 superior mesenteric vein

11　肠系膜上动脉 superior mesenteric artery

12　腹主动脉 abdominal aorta　　　　13　左肾 left kidney

14　右肾 right kidney　　　　　　　15　右膈脚 right crus of diaphragm

16　下腔静脉 inferior vena cava

17　胰钩突 uncinate process of pancreas　　18　胰头 head of pancreas

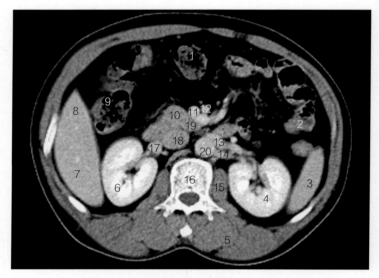

图 1-12　经肾门上份的横断层 CT 图像

1	横结肠 transverse colon	2	结肠左曲 left colic flexure
3	脾 spleen	4	左肾 left kidney
5	竖脊肌 erector spinae	6	右肾 right kidney

7　肝右后叶 right posterior lobe of liver

8　肝右前叶 right anterior lobe of liver

9　十二指肠降部 descending part of duodenum

10　胰头 head of pancreas

11　肠系膜上静脉 superior mesenteric vein

12　肠系膜上动脉 superior mesenteric artery

13	左肾静脉 left renal vein	14	左肾动脉 left renal artery

15　腰大肌 psoas major

16　第 1 腰椎椎体 body of 1st lumbar vertebrae

17	右肾静脉 right renal vein	18	下腔静脉 inferior vena cava
19	胰钩突 uncinate process of pancreas	20	腹主动脉 abdominal aorta

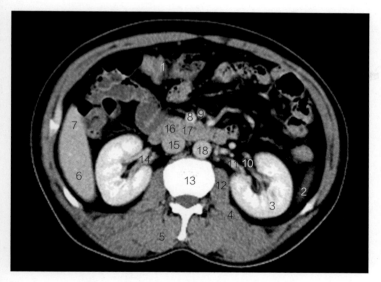

图 1-13　经肾门中份的横断层 CT 图像

1　横结肠 transverse colon

2　脾 spleen

3　左肾 left kidney

4　腰方肌 quadratus lumborum

5　竖脊肌 erector spinae

6　肝右后叶 right posterior lobe of liver

7　肝右前叶 right anterior lobe of liver

8　肠系膜上静脉 superior mesenteric vein

9　肠系膜上动脉 superior mesenteric artery

10　左肾静脉 left renal vein

11　左肾动脉 left renal artery

12　腰大肌 psoas major

13　第 1 腰椎间盘 1st lumbar intervertebral disc

14　右肾动脉、静脉 right renal artery and vein

15　下腔静脉 inferior vena cava

16　胰头 head of pancreas

17　胰钩突 uncinate process of pancreas

18　腹主动脉 abdominal aorta

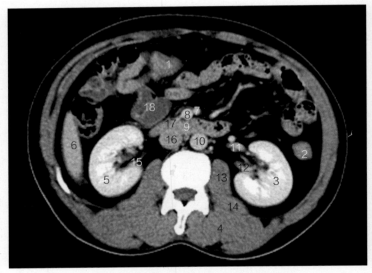

图 1-14　经肾门中份的横断层 CT 图像

1　横结肠 transverse colon	2　降结肠 descending colon
3　左肾 left kidney	4　竖脊肌 erector spinae
5　右肾 right kidney	6　肝 liver
7　肠系膜上动脉 superior mesenteric artery	
8　肠系膜上静脉 superior mesenteric vein	
9　胰钩突 uncinate process of pancreas	10　腹主动脉 abdominal aorta
11　左肾静脉 left renal vein	12　左肾动脉 left renal artery
13　腰大肌 psoas major	14　腰方肌 quadratus lumborum
15　右肾动脉 right renal artery	16　下腔静脉 inferior vena cava
17　胰头 head of pancreas	
18　十二指肠降部 descending part of duodenum	

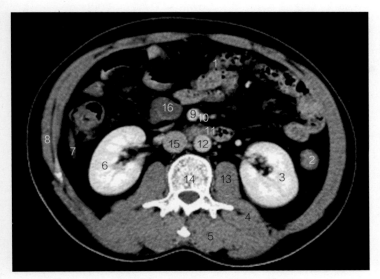

图 1-15 经肾门下份的横断层 CT 图像

1 横结肠 transverse colon	2 降结肠 descending colon
3 左肾 left kidney	4 腰方肌 quadratus lumborum
5 竖脊肌 erector spinae	6 右肾 right kidney

7 肝 liver

8 腹外斜肌 obliquus externus abdominis

9 肠系膜上静脉 superior mesenteric vein

10 肠系膜上动脉 superior mesenteric artery

11 十二指肠水平部 horizontal part of duodenum

12 腹主动脉 abdominal aorta	13 腰大肌 psoas major

14 第 2 腰椎椎体 body of 2nd lumbar vertebrae

15 下腔静脉 inferior vena cava

16 十二指肠降部 descending part of duodenum

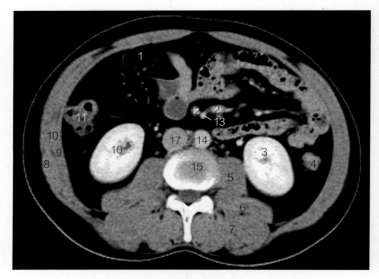

图 1-16　经第二腰椎间盘的横断层 CT 图像

1　横结肠 transverse colon

2　空肠静脉 jejunal vein

3　左肾 left kidney

4　降结肠 descending colon

5　腰大肌 psoas major

6　腰方肌 quadratus lumborum

7　竖脊肌 erector spinae

8　腹外斜肌 obliquus externus abdominis

9　腹横肌 transversus abdominis

10　腹内斜肌 obliquus internus abdominis

11　结肠右曲 right colic flexure

12　肠系膜上静脉 superior mesenteric vein

13　肠系膜上动脉 superior mesenteric artery

14　腹主动脉 abdominal aorta

15　第 2 腰椎间盘 2nd lumbar intervertebral disc

16　右肾 right kidney

17　下腔静脉 inferior vena cava

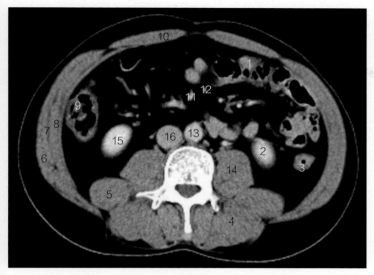

图 1-17　经左肾下极的横断层 CT 图像

1　横结肠 transverse colon　　　　2　左肾 left kidney

3　降结肠 descending colon　　　　4　竖脊肌 erector spinae

5　腰方肌 quadratus lumborum

6　腹外斜肌 obliquus externus abdominis

7　腹内斜肌 obliquus internus abdominis

8　腹横肌 transversus abdominis　　9　升结肠 ascending colon

10　腹直肌 rectus abdominis

11　肠系膜上静脉 superior mesenteric vein

12　肠系膜上动脉 superior mesenteric artery

13　腹主动脉 abdominal aorta　　　14　腰大肌 psoas major

15　右肾 right kidney　　　　　　16　下腔静脉 inferior vena cava

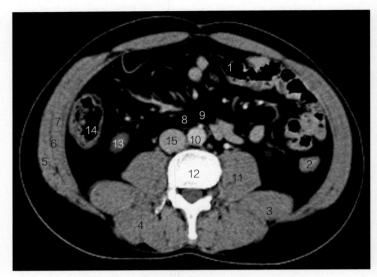

图 1-18　经肠系膜下动脉的横断层 CT 图像

1　横结肠 transverse colon

2　降结肠 descending colon

3　腰方肌 quadratus lumborum

4　竖脊肌 erector spinae

5　腹外斜肌 obliquus externus abdominis

6　腹内斜肌 obliquus internus abdominis

7　腹横肌 transversus abdominis

8　肠系膜上静脉 superior mesenteric vein

9　肠系膜下动脉 inferior mesenteric artery

10　腹主动脉 abdominal aorta

11　腰大肌 psoas major

12　第 3 腰椎椎体 body of 3rd lumbar vertebrae

13　右肾 right kidney

14　升结肠 ascending colon

15　下腔静脉 inferior vena cava

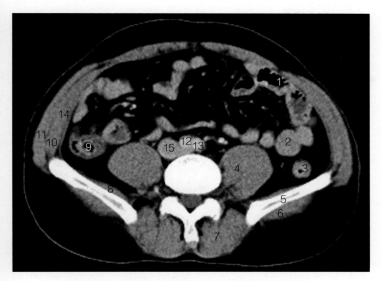

图 1-19　经腹主动脉分叉处的横断层 CT 图像

1　横结肠 transverse colon	2　空肠 jejunum
3　降结肠 descending colon	4　腰大肌 psoas major
5　髂骨翼 ala of ilium	6　臀中肌 gluteus medius
7　竖脊肌 erector spinae	8　髂肌 iliacus
9　升结肠 ascending colon	
10　腹内斜肌 obliquus internus abdominis	
11　腹外斜肌 obliquus externus abdominis	
12　右髂总动脉 right common iliac artery	
13　左髂总动脉 left common iliac artery	
14　腹横肌 transversus abdominis	15　下腔静脉 inferior vena cava

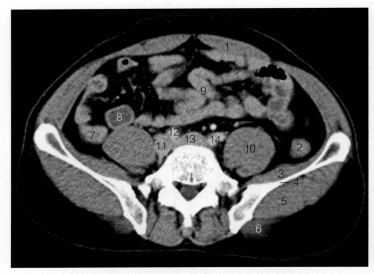

图 1-20　经下腔静脉合成处的横断层 CT 图像

1　腹直肌 rectus abdominis

2　降结肠 descending colon

3　髂肌 iliacus

4　髂骨翼 ala of ilium

5　臀中肌 gluteus medius

6　臀大肌 gluteus maximus

7　盲肠 cecum

8　回肠 ileum

9　空肠 jejunum

10　腰大肌 psoas major

11　右髂总静脉 right common iliac vein

12　右髂总动脉 right common iliac artery

13　左髂总静脉 left common iliac vein

14　左髂总动脉 left common iliac artery

第二章 腹部矢状断层 CT 图像

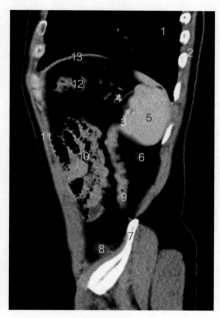

图 2-1　经降结肠的矢状断层 CT 图像

1　左肺上叶 superior lobe of left lung

2　背阔肌 latissimus dorsi

3　脾裸区 bare area of spleen

4　脾静脉 splenic vein

5　脾 spleen

6　左肾 left kidney

7　髂骨 ilium

8　乙状结肠 sigmoid colon

9　降结肠 descending colon

10　回肠 ileum

11　腹外斜肌 obliquus externus abdominis

12　横结肠 transverse colon

13　膈 diaphragm

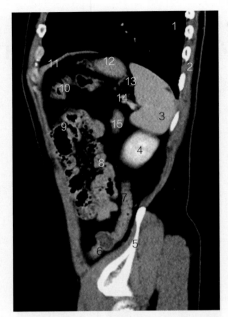

图 2-2 经左肾外侧份的矢状断层 CT 图像

1 左肺上叶 superior lobe of left lung

2 背阔肌 latissimus dorsi

3 脾 spleen

4 左肾 left kidney

5 髂骨 ilium

6 乙状结肠 sigmoid colon

7 降结肠 descending colon

8 空肠 jejunum

9 回肠 ileum

10 横结肠 transverse colon

11 膈 diaphragm

12 胃底 fundus of stomach

13 胃脾隐窝 gastrosplenic recess

14 脾静脉 splenic vein

15 胰尾 tail of pancreas

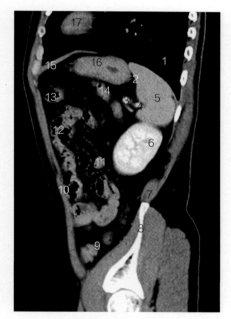

图 2-3 经胰尾的矢状断层 CT 图像

1 左肺下叶 inferior lobe of left lung	2 胃脾隐窝 gastrosplenic recess
3 脾静脉 splenic vein	4 脾动脉 splenic artery
5 脾 spleen	6 左肾 left kidney
7 腰方肌 quadratus lumborum	8 髂骨 ilium
9 乙状结肠 sigmoid colon	10 腹直肌 rectus abdominis
11 空肠 jejunum	12 回肠 ileum
13 横结肠 transverse colon	14 胰尾 tail of pancreas
15 膈 diaphragm	16 胃底 fundus of stomach
17 左心室 left ventricle	

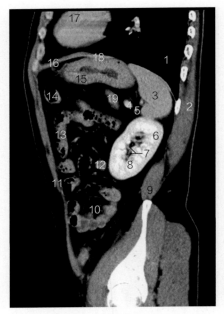

图 2-4　经脾门的矢状断层 CT 图像

1　左肺下叶 inferior lobe of left lung

2　竖脊肌 erector spinae

3　脾 spleen

4　脾静脉 splenic vein

5　脾动脉 splenic artery

6　左肾 left kidney

7　左肾动、静脉 left renal artery and vein

8　肾锥体 renal pyramid

9　腰方肌 quadratus lumborum

10　空肠动脉 jejunal artery

11　腹直肌 rectus abdominis

12　空肠 jejunum

13　回肠 ileum

14　横结肠 transverse colon

15　胃体 body of stomach

16　膈 diaphragm

17　左心室 left ventricle

18　肝左外叶 left lateral lobe of liver

19　胰尾 tail of pancreas

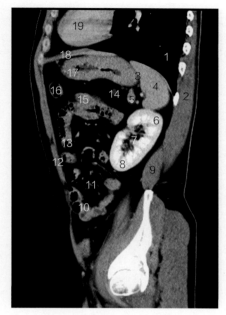

图 2-5 经左肾窦的矢状断层 CT 图像

1 左肺下叶 inferior lobe of left lung

2 竖脊肌 erector spinae

3 胃脾隐窝 gastrosplenic recess

4 脾 spleen

5 脾静脉 splenic vein

6 左肾 left kidney

7 左肾窦 left renal sinus

8 肾锥体 renal pyramid

9 腰方肌 quadratus lumborum

10 乙状结肠 sigmoid colon

11 乙状结肠动脉 sigmoid artery

12 腹直肌 rectus abdominis

13 回肠 ileum

14 胰尾 tail of pancreas

15 空肠 jejunum

16 横结肠 transverse colon

17 胃体 body of stomach

18 膈 diaphragm

19 左心室 left ventricle

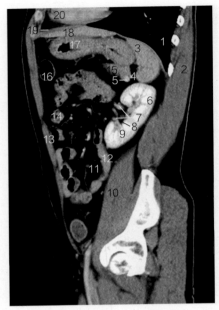

图 2-6 经肝左上角的矢状断层 CT 图像

1 左肺下叶 inferior lobe of left lung	2 竖脊肌 erector spinae
3 脾 spleen	4 脾动脉 splenic artery
5 脾静脉 splenic vein	6 左肾 left kidney
7 左肾动、静脉 left renal artery and vein	8 左肾窦 left renal sinus
9 肾锥体 renal pyramid	10 腰大肌 psoas major
11 空肠动脉 jejunal artery	12 空肠 jejunum
13 腹直肌 rectus abdominis	14 回肠 ileum
15 胰体 body of pancreas	16 横结肠 transverse colon
17 胃体 body of stomach	
18 肝左外叶 left lateral lobe of liver	19 膈 diaphragm
20 左心室 left ventricle	

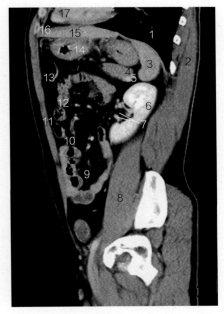

图 2-7　经左肾门的矢状断层 CT 图像

1　左肺下叶 inferior lobe of left lung　　　　2　竖脊肌 erector spinae

3　脾 spleen　　　　4　胰体 body of pancreas

5　脾动、静脉 splenic artery and vein　　　　6　左肾 left kidney

7　左肾动、静脉 left renal artery and vein

8　腰大肌 psoas major　　　　9　空肠动脉 jejunal artery

10　空肠 jejunum　　　　11　腹直肌 rectus abdominis

12　回肠 ileum　　　　13　横结肠 transverse colon

14　胃体 body of stomach

15　肝左外叶 left lateral lobe of liver　　　　16　膈 diaphragm

17　左心室 left ventricle

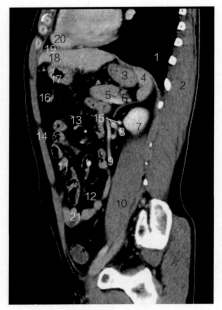

图 2-8 经脾前端的矢状断层 CT 图像

1　左肺下叶 inferior lobe of left lung　　2　竖脊肌 erector spinae

3　胃底和贲门 fundus and cardia of stomach

4　脾 spleen　　5　胰体 body of pancreas

6　脾动、静脉 splenic artery and vein　　7　左肾 left kidney

8　左肾动脉分支 branch of left renal artery

9　肠系膜上静脉 superior mesenteric vein

10　腰大肌 psoas major　　11　回肠 ileum

12　空肠动脉 jejunal artery　　13　空肠 jejunum

14　腹直肌 rectus abdominis

15　肾动、静脉 renal artery and vein　　16　横结肠 transverse colon

17　胃体 body of stomach

18　肝左外叶 left lateral lobe of liver　　19　膈 diaphragm

20　左心室 left ventricle　　21　乙状结肠 sigmoid colon

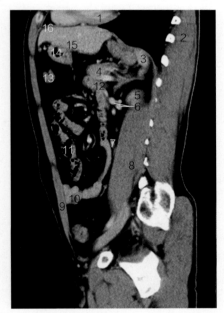

图 2-9 经十二指肠空肠曲的矢状断层 CT 图像

1	左心室 left ventricle	2	竖脊肌 erector spinae
3	脾 spleen	4	胰体 body of pancreas
5	左肾 left kidney		
6	左肾动、静脉 left renal artery and vein		
7	肠系膜上静脉 superior mesenteric vein		
8	腰大肌 psoas major	9	腹直肌 rectus abdominis
10	乙状结肠 sigmoid colon	11	回肠 ileum
12	十二指肠空肠曲 duodenojejunal flexure		
13	横结肠 transverse colon	14	胃体 body of stomach
15	肝左外叶 left lateral lobe of liver	16	膈 diaphragm

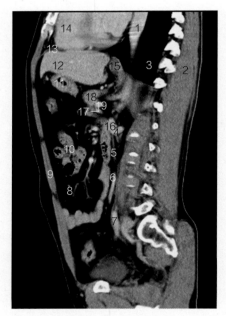

图 2-10　经食管腹段的矢状断层 CT 图像

1　胸主动脉 thoracic aorta
2　竖脊肌 erector spinae
3　左肺下叶 inferior lobe of left lung
4　左肾动脉 left renal artery
5　左睾丸静脉 left testicular vein
6　肠系膜上静脉 superior mesenteric vein
7　左髂总动脉 left common iliac artery
8　空肠动脉 jejunal artery
9　腹直肌 rectus abdominis
10　空肠 jejunum
11　胃体 body of stomach
12　肝左外叶 left lateral lobe of liver
13　膈 diaphragm
14　右心室 right ventricle
15　食管腹段 abdominal part of esophagus
16　左肾静脉 left renal vein
17　脾静脉 splenic vein
18　胰体 body of pancreas
19　脾动脉 splenic artery

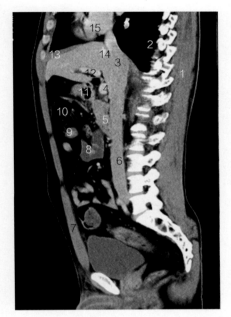

图 2-11 经降主动脉的矢状断层 CT 图像

1	竖脊肌 erector spinae	2	左肺下叶 inferior lobe of left lung
3	胸主动脉 thoracic aorta	4	肝门静脉 hepatic portal vein
5	胰头 head of pancreas	6	腹主动脉 abdomine aorta
7	腹直肌 rectus abdominis	8	回肠 ileum
9	空肠 jejunum	10	横结肠 transverse colon
11	胃体 body of stomach		

12 肝门静脉左支 left hepatic portal vein

13 膈 diaphragm

14	肝中静脉 middle hepatic vein	15	右心房 right atrium

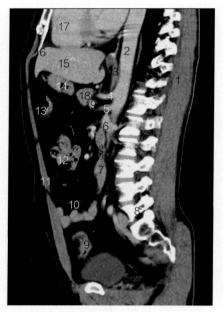

图 2-12　经腹腔干的矢状断层 CT 图像

1　竖脊肌 erector spinae	2　胸主动脉 thoracic aorta
3　食管腹段 abdominal part of esophagus	4　腹腔干 celiac trunk
5　肠系膜上动脉 superior mesenteric artery	
6　左肾静脉 left renal vein	7　腹主动脉 abdominal aorta
8　第 5 腰椎椎体 body of 5th lumbar vertebrae	
9　乙状结肠 sigmoid colon	10　空肠动脉 jejunal artery
11　腹直肌 rectus abdominis	12　空肠 jejunum
13　横结肠 transverse colon	14　胃体 body of stomach
15　肝左外叶 left lateral lobe of liver	16　膈 diaphragm
17　右心室 right ventricle	18　胰体 body of pancreas
19　脾静脉 splenic vein	

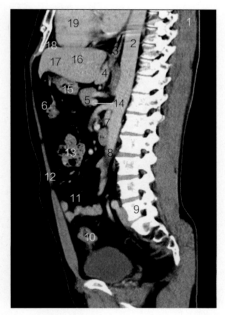

图 2-13 经肠系膜上动脉的矢状断层 CT 图像

1	竖脊肌 erector spinae	2	胸主动脉 thoracic aorta
3	食管腹段 abdominal part of esophagus	4	肝尾状叶 caudate lobe of liver
5	胰体 body of pancreas	6	横结肠 transverse colon
7	左肾静脉 left renal vein	8	腹主动脉 abdominal aorta
9	第 5 腰椎椎体 body of 5th lumbar vertebrae		
10	乙状结肠 sigmoid colon	11	空肠动脉 jejunal artery
12	腹直肌 rectus abdominis	13	空肠 jejunum
14	脾静脉 splenic vein	15	胃体 body of stomach
16	肝门静脉左支 left hepatic poratal vein		
17	肝左外叶 left lateral lobe of liver	18	膈 diaphragm
19	右心室 right ventricle		

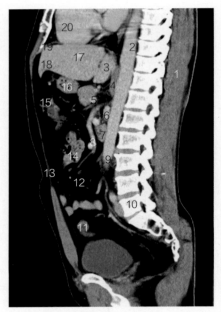

图 2-14　经胃幽门部和肝门静脉左支的矢状断层 CT 图像

1	竖脊肌 erector spinae	2	胸主动脉 thoracic aorta
3	肝尾状叶 caudate lobe of liver		
4	食管腹段 abdominal part of esophagus	5	脾静脉 splenic vein
6	左肾静脉 left renal vein		
7	十二指肠水平部 horizontal part of duodenum		
8	肠系膜上动脉 superior mesenteric artery		
9	腹主动脉 abdominal aorta		
10	第 5 腰椎椎体 body of 5th lumbar vertebrae		
11	乙状结肠 sigmoid colon	12	空肠动脉 jejunal artery
13	白线 white line	14	空肠 jejunum
15	横结肠 transverse colon	16	胃幽门部 pyloric part of stomach
17	肝门静脉左支 left hepatic portal vein		
18	肝左外叶 left lateral lobe of liver	19	膈 diaphragm
20	右心室 right ventricle		

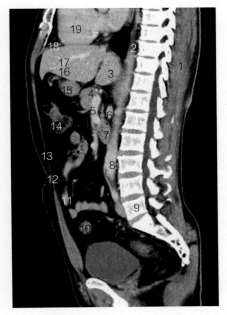

图 2-15　经肠系膜上静脉的矢状断层 CT 图像

1　竖脊肌 erector spinae

2　胸主动脉 thoracic aorta

3　肝尾状叶 caudate lobe of liver

4　胰头 head of pancreas

5　肠系膜上静脉 superior mesenteric vein

6　左肾静脉 left renal vein

7　十二指肠肠水平部 horizontal part of duodenum

8　腹主动脉 abdominal aorta

9　第 5 腰椎椎体 body of 5th lumbar vertebrae

10　乙状结肠 sigmoid colon

11　回肠 ileum

12　脐 umbilical region

13　白线 white line

14　空肠 jejunum

15　胃幽门部 pyloric part of stomach

16　肝左外叶 left lateral lobe of liver

17　肝左静脉 left hepatic vein

18　膈 diaphragm

19　右心室 right ventricle

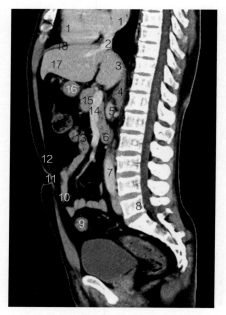

图 2-16   经脐的矢状断层 CT 图像

1　右心室 right ventricle 　　　　　2　下腔静脉 inferior vena cava

3　肝尾状叶 caudate lobe of liver 　　4　右肾上腺 right suprarenal gland

5　左肾静脉 left renal vein

6　十二指肠肠水平部 horizontal part of duodenum

7　腹主动脉 abdominal aorta

8　第 5 腰椎椎体 body of 5th lumbar vertebrae

9　乙状结肠 sigmoid colon 　　　　　10　回肠 ileum

11　脐 umbilical region 　　　　　　12　白线 white line

13　空肠 jejunum

14　肠系膜上静脉 superior mesenteric vein

15　胰头 head of pancreas 　　　　　16　胃幽门部 pyloric part of stomach

17　肝左外叶 left lateral lobe of liver 　18　膈 diaphragm

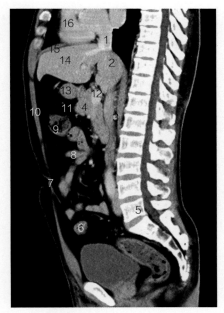

图 2-17　经下腔静脉和肝左静脉的矢状断层 CT 图像

1　下腔静脉 inferior vena cava　　　　2　肝尾状叶 caudate lobe of liver

3　右肾动脉 right renal artery　　　　4　胰头 head of pancreas

5　第 5 腰椎椎体 body of 5th lumbar vertebrae

6　乙状结肠 sigmoid colon　　　　　　7　脐 umbilical region

8　回肠 ileum　　　　　　　　　　　　9　空肠 jejunum

10　腹直肌 rectus abdominis　　　　　11　横结肠 transverse colon

12　肝门静脉 hepatic portal vein　　　13　胃幽门部 pyloric part of stomach

14　肝左外叶 left lateral lobe of liver　15　膈 diaphragm

16　右心室 right ventricle

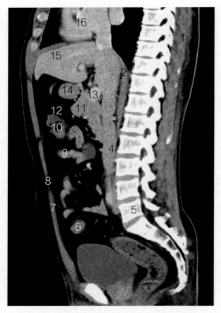

图 2-18　经下腔静脉和肝门静脉的矢状断层 CT 图像

1　竖脊肌 erector spinae	2　膈 diaphragm
3　右肾动脉 right renal artery	4　下腔静脉 inferior vena cava
5　第 5 腰椎椎体 body of 5th lumbar vertebrae	
6　乙状结肠 sigmoid colon	7　腹直肌 rectus abdomimis
8　脐 umbilical region	9　回肠 ileum
10　空肠 jejunum	11　胰头 head of pancreas
12　横结肠 transverse colon	13　肝门静脉 hepatic portal vein
14　胃幽门部 pyloric part of stomach	15　肝左外叶 left lateral lobe of liver
16　右心室 right ventricle	

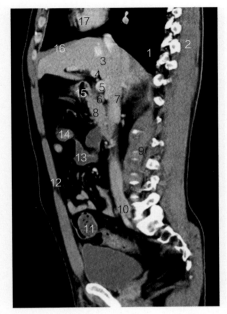

图 2-19   经下腔静脉和肝门静脉左支的矢状断层 CT 图像

1   右肺下叶 inferior lobe of right lung

2   竖脊肌 erector spinae

3   肝左内叶 left medial lobe of liver

4   肝门静脉左支 left hepatic portal vein

5   肝门静脉 hepatic portal vein

6   门腔淋巴结 portocaval lymph node

7   下腔静脉 inferior vena cava

8   胰头 head of pancreas

9   腰大肌 poas major

10   左髂总静脉 left common iliac vein

11   乙状结肠 sigmoid colon

12   腹直肌 rectus abdominis

13   回肠 ileum

14   空肠 jejunum

15   横结肠 transverse colon

16   膈 diaphragm

17   右心房 right atrium

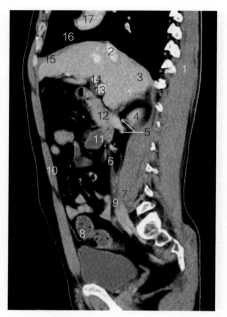

图 2-20　经右肾门内侧份的 CT 矢状断层图像

1　竖脊肌 erector spinae
2　下腔静脉 inferior vena cava
3　肝左内叶 left medial lobe of liver
4　右肾 right kidney
5　右肾动、静脉 right renal artery and vein
6　下腔静脉 inferior vena cava
7　腰大肌 psoas major
8　乙状结肠 sigmoid colon
9　左髂总静脉 left common iliac vein
10　腹直肌 rectus abdominis
11　回肠 ileum
12　胰头 head of pancreas
13　肝门静脉 hepatic portal vein
14　肝门静脉左支 left hepatic portal vein
15　膈 diaphragm
16　右肺下叶 inferior lobe of right lung
17　右心房 right atrium

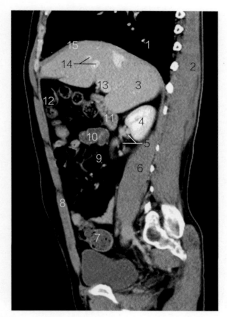

图 2-21 经肝门静脉右支的 CT 矢状断层图像

1 右肺下叶 inferior lobe of right lung 　 2 竖脊肌 erector spinae

3 肝右叶 right lobe of liver 　 4 右肾 right kidney

5 右肾动、静脉 right renal artery and vein

6 腰大肌 psoas major 　 7 乙状结肠 sigmoid colon

8 腹直肌 rectus abdominis 　 9 空肠 jejunum

10 回肠 ileum 　 11 胰头 head of pancreas

12 横结肠 transverse colon

13 肝门静脉右支 right hepatic portal vein

14 肝门静脉左支 left branch of hepatic portal vein

15 膈 diaphragm

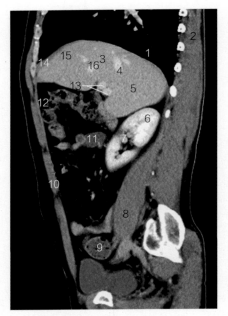

图 2-22 经肝门静脉右支分叉处的矢状断层 CT 图像

1　右肺下叶 inferior lobe of right lung	2　竖脊肌 erector spinae
3　肝右前叶 right anterior lobe of liver	4　肝右静脉 right hepatic vein
5　肝右后叶 right posterior lobe of liver	6　右肾 right kidney
7　右肾静脉 right renal vein	8　腰大肌 psoas major
9　乙状结肠 sigmoid colon	10　腹直肌 rectus abdominis
11　回肠 ileum	12　横结肠 transverse colon

13　肝门静脉右支 right hepatic portal vein

14　膈 diaphragm

15　肝左内叶 left medial lobe of liver

16　肝中静脉 middle hepatic vein

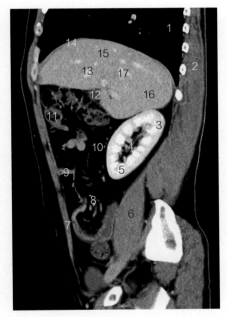

图 2-23　经右肾窦的矢状断层 CT 图像

1	右肺下叶 inferior lobe of right lung	2	竖脊肌 erector spinae
3	右肾 right kidney	4	右肾静脉 right renal vein
5	肾锥体 renal pyramid	6	腰大肌 psoas major
7	腹直肌 rectus abdominis	8	回肠 ileum
9	大网膜 greater omentum	10	升结肠 ascending colon
11	结肠右曲 right colic flexure	12	胆囊 gallbladder

13　肝门静脉左内支 left medial branch of hepatic portal vein

14　膈 diaphragm

15　肝右前叶 right anterior lobe of liver

16　肝右后叶 right poterior lobe of liver

17　肝门静脉右前支 right anterior branch of hepatic portal vein

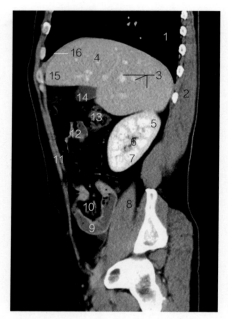

图 2-24　经胆囊和肝门静脉右前支的矢状断层 CT 图像

1　右肺下叶 inferior lobe of right lung

2　竖脊肌 erector spinae

3　肝门静脉右前支 right anterior branch of hepatic portal vein

4　肝右前叶 right anterior lobe of liver

5　右肾 right kidney

6　肾窦 renal sinus

7　肾锥体 renal pyramid

8　腰大肌 psoas major

9　乙状结肠 sigmoid colon

10　乙状结肠动脉 sigmoid artery

11　腹直肌 rectus abdominis

12　回肠 ileum

13　升结肠 ascending colon

14　胆囊 gallbladder

15　肝左内叶 left medial lobe of liver

16　膈 diaphragm

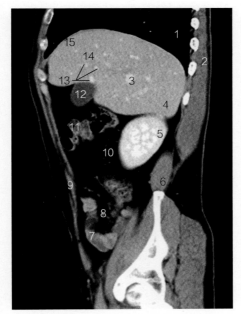

图 2-25　经胆囊右份的矢状断层 CT 图像

1　右肺下叶 inferior lobe of right lung　　　2　背阔肌 latissimus dorsi

3　肝门静脉右前上支 right anterosuperior branch of hepatic portal vein

4　肝右后叶 right posterior lobe of liver　　5　右肾 right kidney

6　腰方肌 quadratus lumborum　　　　　　7　乙状结肠 sigmoid colon

8　乙状结肠动脉 sigmoid artery　　　　　　9　腹直肌 rectus abdominis

10　升结肠 ascending colon　　　　　　　　11　回肠 ileum

12　胆囊 gallbladder

13　肝门静脉左内支 left medial branch of hepatic portal vein

14　肝右前叶 right anterior lobe of liver　　15　膈 diaphragm

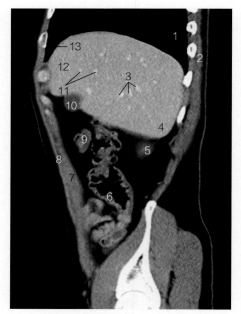

图 2-26 经右肾外侧的矢状断层 CT 图像

1 右肺下叶 inferior lobe of lung 　　2 背阔肌 latissimus dorsi

3 肝门静脉右后下支 right posteroinferior branch of hepatic portal vein

4 肝右后叶 right posterior lobe of liver 　5 右肾 right kidney

6 升结肠 ascending colon 　　7 腹横肌 transversus abdominis

8 腹直肌 rectus abdomimis 　　9 回肠 ileum

10 胆囊 gallbladder

11 肝门静脉右前上支 right anterosuperior branch of hepatic portal vein

12 肝右前叶 right anterior lobe of liver 　13 膈 diaphragm

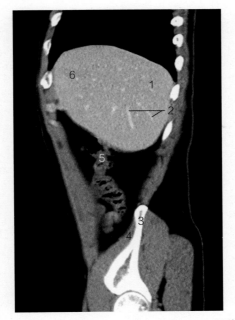

图 2-27 经肝胆囊窝右侧的矢状断层 CT 图像

1 肝右后叶 right posterior lobe of liver

2 肝门静脉右后下支 right posteroinferior branch of hepatic portal vein

3 髂骨翼 ala of ilium　　　　4 髂肌 iliacus

5 升结肠 ascending colon　　　6 肝右前叶 right anterior lobe of liver

第三章 腹部冠状断层 CT 图像

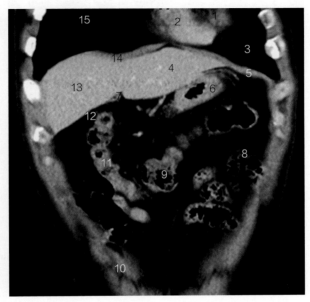

图 3-1 经肝圆韧带的冠状断层 CT 图像

1 左心室 left ventricle
2 右心室 right ventricle
3 左肺上叶 superior lobe of left lung
4 肝左外叶 left lateral lobe of liver
5 膈 diaphragm
6 胃体 body of stomach
7 肝圆韧带 ligamentum teres hepatis
8 降结肠 descending colon
9 回肠 ileum
10 腹直肌 rectus abdominis
11 升结肠 ascending colon
12 右肝下间隙 right subhepatic space
13 肝左内叶 left medial lobe of liver
14 肝镰状韧带 falciform ligament of liver
15 右肺中叶 middle lobe of right lung

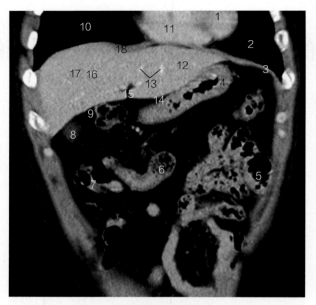

图 3-2 经胆囊底的冠状断层 CT 图像

1 左心室 left ventricle   2 左肺上叶 superior lobe of left lung

3 膈 diaphragm   4 胃体 body of stomach

5 降结肠 descending colon   6 回肠 ileum

7 升结肠 ascending colon   8 胆囊底 fundus of gallbladder

9 右肝下间隙 right subhepatic space

10 右肺中叶 middle lobe of right lung

11 右心室 right ventricle   12 肝左外叶 left lateral lobe of liver

13 肝门静脉左外下支 left lateroinferior branch of hepatic portal vein

14 左肝下前间隙 anterior left subhepatic space

15 肝圆韧带裂 fissure for ligamentum teres hepatis

16 肝中静脉属支 tributaries of middle hepatic vein

17 肝左内叶 left medial lobe of liver

18 肝裸区 bare area of liver

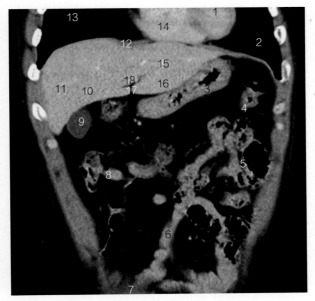

图 3-3　经肝左静脉下根和胆囊底的冠状断层 CT 图像

1　左心室 left ventricle
2　左肺上叶 superior lobe of left lung

3　胃体 body of stomach
4　横结肠 transverse colon

5　降结肠 descending colon
6　回肠 ileum

7　腹直肌 rectus abdominis
8　升结肠 ascending colon

9　胆囊底 fundus of gallbladder

10　肝中静脉属支 tributaries of middle hepatic vein

11　肝右前叶 right anterior lobe of liver
12　肝裸区 bare area of liver

13　右肺中叶 middle lobe of right lung
14　右心室 right ventricle

15　肝左静脉下根属支 tributary of inferior root of left hepatic vein

16　肝左外叶 left lateral lobe of liver

17　肝圆韧带裂 fissure for ligamentum teres hepacis

18　肝门静脉左支囊部 sac part of left hepatic portal vein

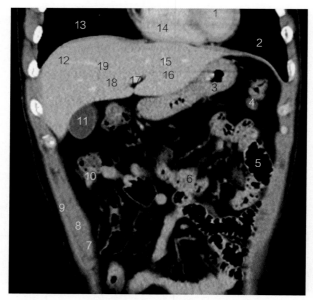

图 3-4　经肝门静脉左支囊部的冠状断层 CT 图像

1　左心室 left ventricle

2　左肺上叶 superior lobe of left lung

3　胃体 body of stomach

4　横结肠 transverse colon

5　降结肠 descending colon

6　回肠 ileum

7　腹横肌 transversus abdominis

8　腹内斜肌 obliquus internus abdominis

9　腹外斜肌 obliquus externus abdominis

10　升结肠 ascending colon

11　胆囊体 body of gallbladder

12　肝右前叶 right anterior lobe of liver

13　右肺 right lung

14　右心室 right ventricle

15　肝左静脉下根 inferior root of left hepatic vein

16　肝左外叶 left lateral lobe of liver

17　肝门静脉左支囊部 sac part of left hepatic portal vein

18　肝左内叶 left medial lobe of liver

19　肝中静脉属支 tributaries of middle hepatic vein

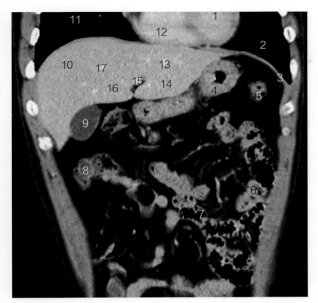

图 3-5　经肝门静脉左支矢状部的冠状断层 CT 图像

1　左心室 left ventricle
2　左肺上叶 superior lobe of left lung
3　膈 diaphragm
4　胃体 body of stomach
5　横结肠 transverse colon
6　降结肠 descending colon
7　空肠 jejunum
8　升结肠 ascending colon
9　胆囊体 body of gallbladder
10　肝右前叶 right anterior lobe of liver
11　右肺 right lung
12　右心室 right ventricle
13　肝左静脉下根 inferior root of left hepatic vein
14　肝左外叶 left lateral lobe of liver
15　肝门静脉左支矢状部 sagittal part of left hepatic portal vein
16　肝左内叶 left medial lobe of liver
17　肝中静脉属支 tributaries of middle hepatic vein

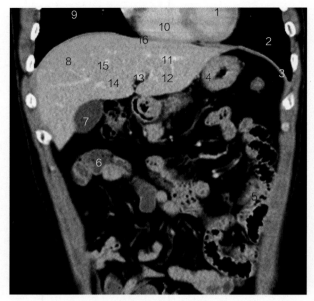

图 3-6　经肝门静脉左支角部的冠状断层 CT 图像

1　左心室 left ventricle

2　左肺上叶 superior lobe of left lung

3　膈 diaphragm

4　胃体 body of stomach

5　降结肠 descending colon

6　横结肠 transverse colon

7　胆囊体 body of gallbladder

8　肝右前叶 right anterior lobe of liver

9　右肺下叶 inferior lobe of right lung

10　右心室 right ventricle

11　肝左静脉属支 tributaries of left hepatic vein

12　肝左外叶 left lateral lobe of liver

13　肝门静脉左支角部 angular part of left hepatic portal vein

14　肝左内叶 left medial lobe of liver

15　肝中静脉属支 tributaries of middle hepatic vein

16　肝裸区 bare area of liver

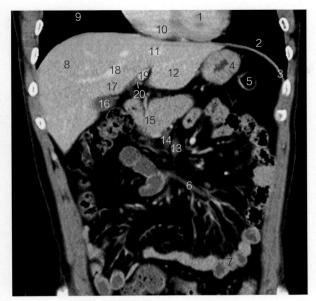

图 3-7　经肝门静脉左支横部的冠状断层 CT 图像

1　左心室 left ventricle

2　左肺 left lung

3　膈 diaphragm

4　胃体 body of stomach

5　横结肠 transverse colon

6　空肠静脉 jejunal vein

7　空肠 jejunum

8　肝右前叶 right anterior lobe of liver

9　右肺下叶 inferior lobe of right lung

10　右心室 right ventricle

11　肝左静脉 left hepatic vein

12　肝左外叶 left lateral lobe of liver

13　肠系膜上动脉 superior mesenteric artery

14　肠系膜上静脉 superior mesenteric vein

15　胰头 head of pancreas

16　胆囊体 body of gallbladder

17　肝左内叶 left medial lobe of liver

18　肝中静脉 middle hepatic vein

19　肝门静脉左支横部 transverse part of left hepatic portal vein

20　小网膜 lesser omentum

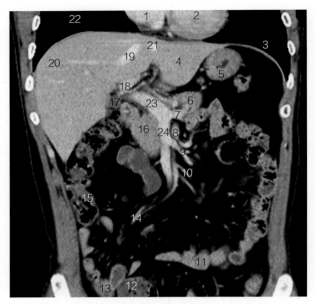

图 3-8　经肝门静脉合成处的冠状断层 CT 图像

1	右心室 right ventricle	2	左心室 left ventricle
3	左肺 left lung	4	肝左外叶 left lateral lobe of liver
5	胃体 body of stomach	6	胰体 body of pancreas
7	脾静脉 splenic vein		
8	肠系膜上动脉 superior mesenteric vein	9	空肠静脉 jejunal vein
10	空肠动脉 jejunal artery	11	空肠 jejunum
12	回肠 ileum	13	盲肠 cecum
14	回结肠动脉 ileocolic artery	15	升结肠 ascending colon
16	胰头 head of pancreas	17	胆囊颈 neck of gallbladder
18	肝门静脉左支横部 transverse part of left hepatic portal vein		
19	肝中静脉 middle hepatic vein		
20	肝右前叶 right anterior lobe of liver	21	肝左静脉 left hepatic vein
22	右肺下叶 inferior lobe of right lung	23	肝门静脉 hepatic portal vein
24	肠系膜上静脉 superior mesenteric vein		

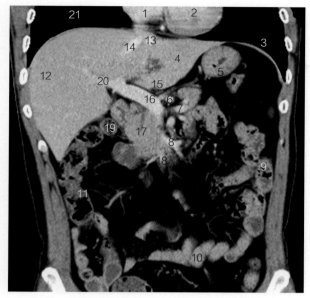

图 3-9　经肝门静脉主干的冠状断层 CT 图像

1	右心房 right atrium	2	左心室 left ventricle
3	左肺 left lung	4	肝左外叶 left lateral lobe of liver
5	胃体 body of stomach	6	肝固有动脉 proper hepatic artery
7	脾静脉 splenic vein		
8	肠系膜上动脉 superior mesenteric artery		
9	降结肠 descending colon	10	空肠 jejunum
11	升结肠 ascending colon	12	肝右前叶 right anterior lobe of liver
13	肝左静脉 left hepatic vein	14	肝中静脉 middle hepatic vein
15	肝尾状叶 caudate lobe of liver		
16	肝门静脉主干 trunk of hepatic portal vein		
17	胰头 head of pancreas		
18	肠系膜上静脉 superior mesenteric vein		
19	十二指肠降部 descending part of duodenum		
20	肝门静脉右支 right hepatic portal vein		
21	右肺下叶 inferior lobe of right lung		

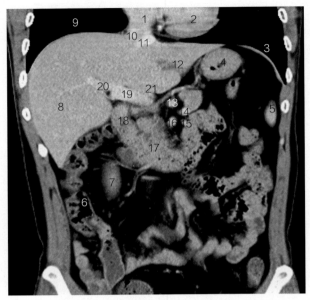

图 3-10　经肝门静脉右前支的冠状断层 CT 图像

1	右心房 right atrium	2	左心室 left ventricle
3	左肺 left lung	4	胃体 body of stomach
5	脾 spleen	6	升结肠 ascending colon
7	右肾 right kidney	8	肝右前叶 right anterior lobe of liver

9　右肺下叶 inferior lobe of right lung

10　肝中静脉 middle hepatic vein　　11　肝左静脉 left hepatic vein

12　肝左外叶 left lateral lobe of liver

13　肝固有动脉 proper hepatic artery

14　脾静脉 splenic vein　　15　肠系膜下静脉 inferior mesenteric vein

16　肠系膜上动脉 superior mesenteric artery

17　胰体 body of pancreas　　18　胰头 head of pancreas

19　肝门静脉 hepatic portal vein

20　肝门静脉右前支 right anterior branch of hepatic portal vein

21　肝尾状叶 caudate lobe of liver

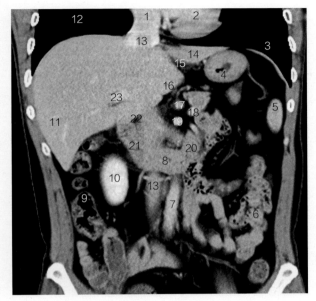

图 3-11　经网膜孔的冠状断层 CT 图像

1　右心房 right atrium	2　左心室 left ventricle
3　左肺下叶 inferior lobe of left lung	4　胃体 body of stomach
5　脾 spleen	6　降结肠 descending colon
7　腹主动脉 abdominal aorta	8　胰颈 neck of pancreas
9　升结肠 ascending colon	10　右肾 right kidney
11　肝右前叶 right anterior lobe of liver	
12　右肺下叶 inferior lobe of right lung	13　下腔静脉 inferior vena cava
14　肝左外叶 left lateral lobe of liver	15　小网膜 lesser omentum
16　肝尾状叶 caudate lobe of liver	17　肝总动脉 common hepatic artery
18　脾静脉 splenic vein	
19　肠系膜上动脉 superior mesenteric artery	
20　胰体 body of pancreas	21　胰头 head of pancreas
22　网膜孔 omental foramen	
23　肝门静脉右后下支 right posteroinferior branch of hepatic portal vein	

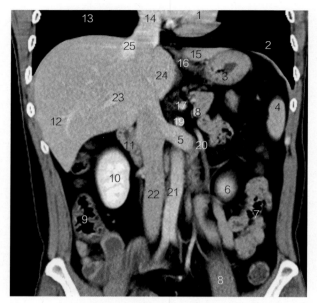

图 3-12   经下腔静脉前份及左肾静脉的冠状断层 CT 图像

1	左心室 left ventricle	2	左肺下叶 inferior lobe of left lung
3	胃体 body of stomach	4	脾 spleen
5	左肾静脉 left renal vein	6	左肾 left kidney
7	降结肠 descending colon	8	腰大肌 psoas major
9	升结肠 ascending colon	10	右肾 right kidney
11	胰头 head of pancreas	12	肝右前叶 right anterior lobe of liver
13	右肺下叶 inferior lobe of right lung		
14	右心房 right atrium	15	肝左外叶 left lateral lobe of liver
16	小网膜 lesser omentum	17	肝总动脉 common hepatic artery
18	脾静脉 splenic vein		
19	肠系膜上动脉 superior mesenteric artery		
20	肠系膜下静脉 inferior mesenteric vein		
21	腹主动脉 abdominal aorta	22	下腔静脉 inferior vena cava
23	肝门静脉右后下支 right posteroinferior branch of hepatic portal vein		
24	肝尾状叶 caudate lobe of liver	25	肝右静脉 right hepatic vein

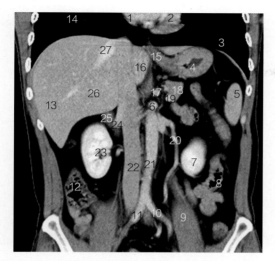

图 3-13　经下腔静脉中份的冠状断层 CT 图像

1　右心房 right atrium　　　　2　左心室 left ventricle
3　左肺下叶 inferior lobe of left lung
4　胃体 body of stomach　　5　脾 spleen
6　肠系膜上动脉 superior mesenteric artery
7　左肾 left kidney　　　　8　降结肠 descending colon
9　腰大肌 psoas major　　　10　左髂总动脉 left common iliac artery
11　右髂总动脉 right common iliac artery
12　升结肠 ascending colon　13　肝右前叶 right anterior lobe of liver
14　右肺下叶 inferior lobe of right lung
15　食管腹段 abdominal part of esophagus
16　肝尾状叶 caudate lobe of liver
17　腹腔干 celiac trunk　　　18　胰体 body of pancreas
19　脾静脉 splenic vein　　　20　肠系膜下静脉 inferior mesenteric vein
21　腹主动脉 abdominal aorta　22　下腔静脉 inferior vena cava
23　右肾 right kidney　　　　24　右肾静脉 right renal vein
25　胰头 head of pancreas
26　肝门静脉右后下支 right posteroinferior branch of hepatic portal vein
27　肝右静脉 right hepatic vein

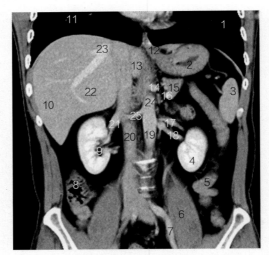

图 3-14 经下腔静脉后份及肝右静脉的冠状断层 CT 图像

1 左肺下叶 inferior lobe of left lung	2 胃 stomach
3 脾 spleen	4 左肾 left kidney
5 降结肠 descending colon	6 腰大肌 psoas major
7 左髂总动脉 left common iliac artery	8 升结肠 ascending colon

9 右肾 right kidney

10 肝右后叶 right posterior lobe of liver

11 右肺下叶 inferior lobe of right lung

12 食管腹段 abdominal part of esophagus

13 肝尾状叶 caudate lobe of liver	14 腹腔干 celiac trunk
15 胰体 body of pancreas	16 脾静脉 splenic vein
17 左肾动脉 left renal artery	18 左肾静脉 left renal vein
19 腹主动脉 abdominal aorta	20 下腔静脉 inferior vena cava

21 右肾静脉 right renal vein

22 肝门静脉右后下支 right posteroinferior branch of hepatic portal vein

23 肝右静脉 right hepatic vein

24 肠系膜上动脉 superior mesenteric artery

25 右肾动脉 right renal artery

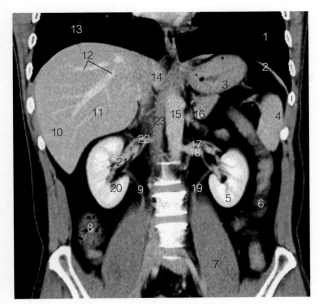

图 3-15 经左、右肾门前份的冠状断层 CT 图像

1 左肺下叶 inferior lobe of left lung 2 膈 diaphragm

3 胃 stomach 4 脾 spleen

5 左肾 left kidney 6 降结肠 descending colon

7 腰大肌 psoas major 8 升结肠 ascending colon

9 右输尿管 right ureter

10 肝右后叶 right posterior lobe of liver

11 肝门静脉右后下支 right posteroinferior branch of hepatic portal vein

12 肝右静脉属支 tributaries of rgiht hepatic vein

13 右肺下叶 inferior lobe of right lung 14 肝尾状叶 caudate lobe of liver

15 腹主动脉 abdominal aorta 16 脾静脉 splenic vein

17 左肾动脉 left renal artery 18 左肾静脉 left renal vein

19 左输尿管 left ureter 20 右肾 right kidney

21 右肾静脉 right renal vein 22 右肾动脉 right renal artery

23 下腔静脉 inferior vena cava

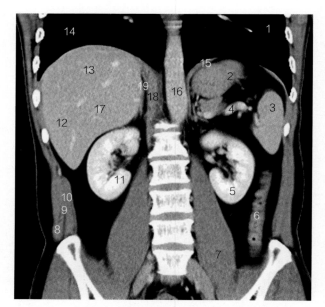

图3-16 经左、右肾门后份的冠状断层CT图像

1 左肺下叶 inferior lobe of left lung	2 胃 stomach
3 脾 spleen	4 脾静脉 splenic vein
5 左肾 left kidney	6 降结肠 descending colon
7 腰大肌 psoas major	
8 腹外斜肌 obliquus externus abdominis	
9 腹内斜肌 obliquus internus abdominis	
10 腹横机 transversus abdominis	11 右肾 right kidney
12 肝右后叶 right posterior lobe of liver	
13 肝右静脉属支 tributaries of right hepatic vein	
14 右肺下叶 inferior lobe of right lung	15 膈 diaphragm
16 腹主动脉 abdominal aorta	
17 肝门静脉右后下支 right posteroinferior branch of hepatic portal vein	
18 右膈脚 right crus of diaphragm	19 肝裸区 bare area of liver

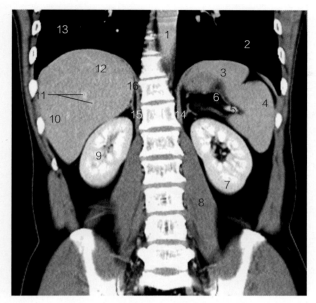

图 3-17 经左、右肾窦后份和脾门的冠状断层 CT 图像

1　胸主动脉 thoracic aorta　　　　　2　左肺下叶 inferior lobe of left lung

3　胃 stomach　　　　　　　　　　4　脾 spleen

5　脾静脉 splenic vein　　　　　　　6　脾门 splenic hilum

7　左肾 left kidney　　　　　　　　　8　腰大肌 psoas major

9　右肾 right kidney

10　肝右后叶 right posterior lobe of liver

11　肝门静脉右后下支 right posteroinferior branch of hepatic portal vein

12　肝右静脉属支 tributaries of right hepatic vein

13　右肺下叶 inferior lobe of right lung　　14　左膈脚 left crus of diaphragm

15　右膈脚 right crus of diaphragm　　　16　肝裸区 bare area of liver

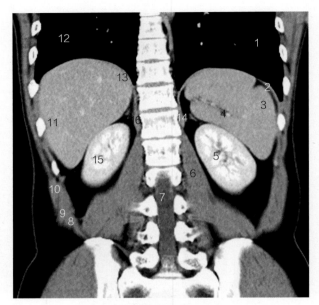

图 3-18　经马尾和脾门层的冠状断层 CT 图像

1　左肺下叶 inferior lobe of left lung	2　膈 diaphragm
3　脾 spleen	4　脾门 splenic hilum
5　左肾 left kidney	6　腰大肌 psoas major
7　马尾 cauda equina	8　腹横肌 transversus abdominis

9　腹内斜肌 obliquus internus abdominis

10　腹外斜肌 obliquus externus abdominis

11　肝右后叶 right posterior lobe of liver

12　右肺下叶 inferior lobe of right lung	13　肝裸区 bare area of liver
14　左膈脚 left crus of diaphragm	15　右肾 right kidney

16　右膈脚 right crus of diaphragm

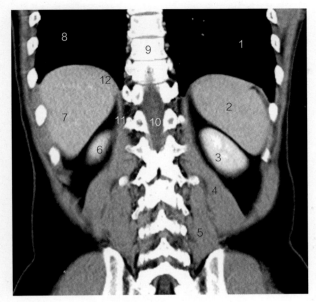

图 3-19　经脊髓的冠状断层 CT 图像

1　左肺下叶 inferior lobe of left lung　　　2　脾 spleen

3　左肾 left kidney　　　4　腰大肌 psoas major

5　竖脊肌 erector spinae　　　6　右肾 right kidney

7　肝右后叶 right posterior lobe of liver

8　右肺下叶 inferior lobe of right lung

9　第 10 胸椎椎体 body of 10th thoracic vertebrae

10　马尾 cauda equina　　　11　右膈脚 right crus of diaphragm

12　肝裸区 bare area of liver

第四章 腹部横断层 MR 图像

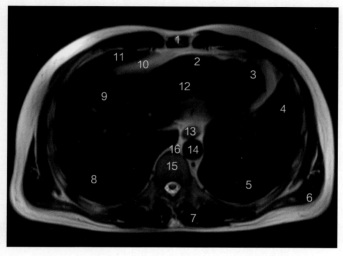

图 4-1 经膈右穹隆的横断层 MR T₂ 加权图像

1	胸骨体 body of sternum	2	右心室 right ventricle
3	左心室 left ventricle	4	左肺上叶 superior lobe of left lung
5	左肺下叶 inferior lobe of left lung	6	背阔肌 latissimus dorsi
7	竖脊肌 erector spinae		
8	右肺下叶 inferior lobe of right lung	9	肝右叶 right lobe of liver
10	膈 diaphragm		
11	左肺中叶 middle lobe of left lung	12	右心房 right atrium
13	食管 esophagus	14	胸主动脉 thoracic aorta
15	第 9 胸椎椎体 body of 9th thoracic vertebrae		
16	奇静脉 azygos vein		

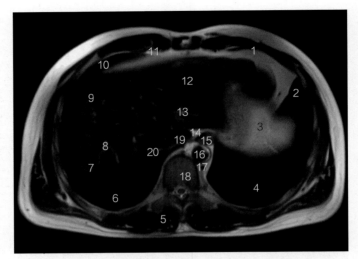

图 4-2 经食管裂孔的横断层 MR T₂ 加权图像

1 肋纵隔隐窝 costomediastinal recess   2 左肺上叶 superior lobe of left lung

3 胃底 fundus of stomach   4 左肺下叶 inferior lobe of left lung

5 竖脊肌 erector spinae

6 右肺下叶 inferior lobe of right lung

7 肝右后叶 right posterior lobe of liver

8 肝门静脉右前上支 right anterosuperior branch of hepatic portal vein

9 肝右前叶 right anterior lobe of liver

10 右肺中叶 middle lobe of right lung

11 肝镰状韧带 falciform ligament of liver

12 肝左外叶 left lateral lobe of liver

13 肝门静脉左外上支 left laterosuperior branch of hepatic portal vein

14 静脉韧带裂 fissure for ligamentum venosum

15 食管 esophagus   16 胸主动脉 thoracic aorta

17 半奇静脉 hemiazygos vein

18 第 10 胸椎椎体 body of 10th thoracic vertebrae

19 肝尾状叶 caudate lobe of liver   20 下腔静脉 inferior vena cava

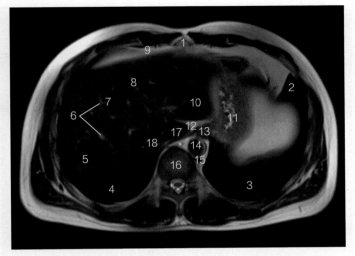

图 4-3　经食管腹段的横断层 MR T$_2$ 加权图像

1　胸骨剑突 xiphoid process of sternum　2　左肺上叶 superior lobe of left lung

3　左肺下叶 inferior lobe of left lung

4　右肺下叶 inferior lobe of right lung

5　肝右后叶 right posterior lobe of liver

6　肝门静脉右前上支 right anterosuperior branch of hepatic portal vein

7　肝右前叶 right anterior lobe of liver　8　肝左内叶 left medial lobe of liver

9　肝镰状韧带 falciform ligament of liver

10　肝左外叶 left lateral lobe of liver　11　胃 stomach

12　静脉韧带裂 fissure for ligamentum venosum

13　食管腹段 abdominal part of esophagus

14　胸主动脉 thoracic aorta　15　半奇静脉 hemiazygos vein

16　第 10 胸椎间盘 10th thoracic intervertebral disc

17　肝尾状叶 caudate lobe of liver　18　下腔静脉 inferior vena cava

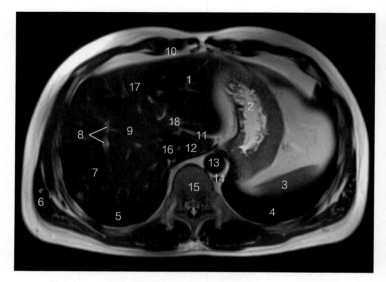

图 4-4　经肝门静脉左支角部的横断层 MR T₂ 加权图像

1　肝左静脉 left hepatic vein

2　胃体 body of stomach

3　脾 spleen

4　左肺下叶 inferior lobe of left lung

5　右肺下叶 inferior lobe of right lung

6　背阔肌 latissimus dorsi

7　肝右后叶 right posterior lobe of liver

8　肝门静脉右前上支 right anterosuperior branch of hepatic portal vein

9　肝中静脉 middle hepatic vein

10　肝镰状韧带 falciform ligament of liver

11　静脉韧带裂 fissure for ligamentum venosum

12　肝尾状叶 caudate lobe of liver

13　胸主动脉 thoracic aorta

14　半奇静脉 hemiazygos vein

15　第 11 胸椎椎体 body of 11th thoracic vertebrae

16　下腔静脉 inferior vena cava

17　肝左内叶 left medial lobe of liver

18　肝门静脉左支角部 angular part of left hepatic portal vein

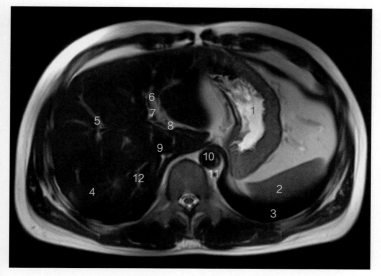

图 4-5 经肝门静脉左支矢状部横断层 MR T$_2$ 加权图像

1　胃体 body of stomach　　　　　2　脾 spleen

3　左肺下叶 inferior lobe of left lung

4　肝右后叶 right posterior lobe of liver

5　肝门静脉右前上支 right anterosuperior branch of hepatic portal vein

6　肝门静脉左支囊部 sac part of left hepatic portal vein

7　肝门静脉左支矢状部 sagittal part of left hepatic portal vein

8　肝门静脉尾状支叶 caudate branch of hepatic portal vein

9　下腔静脉 inferior vena cava　　　　10　胸主动脉 thoracic aorta

11　半奇静脉 hemiazygos vein

12　肝门静脉右后上支 right posterosuperior branch of hepatic portal vein

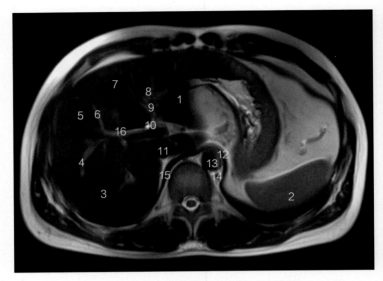

图 4-6 经肝门的横断层 MR T$_2$ 加权图像

1　肝左外叶 left lateral lobe of liver　　　　　2　脾 spleen

3　肝右后叶 right posterior lobe of liver

4　肝门静脉右后支 posterior branch of right hepatic portal vein

5　肝右前叶 right anterior lobe of liver

6　肝门静脉右前支 anterior branch of right hepatic portal vein

7　肝左内叶 left medial lobe of liver

8　肝门静脉左支囊部 sac part of left hepatic portal vein

9　肝门静脉左支矢状部 sagittal part of left hepatic portal vein

10　肝门静脉左支横部 transverse part of left hepatic portal vein

11　下腔静脉 inferior vena cava　　　　12　左膈脚 left crus of diaphragm

13　胸主动脉 thoracic aorta　　　　　　14　半奇静脉 hemiazygos vein

15　右膈脚 right crus of diaphragm

16　肝门静脉右支 right hepatic portal vein

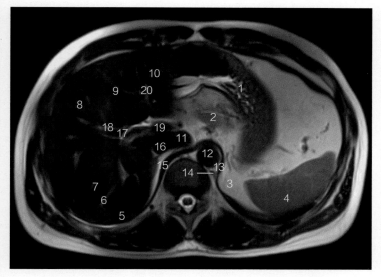

图 4-7　经左肾上腺三角的横断层 MR T$_2$ 加权图像

1　胃体 body of stomach

2　肝胃韧带 hepatogastric ligament

3　左肾上腺三角 left suprarenal gland triangle

4　脾 spleen

5　肝裸区 bare area of liver

6　肝右静脉属支 tributaries of right hepatic vein

7　肝右后叶 right posterior lobe of liver

8　肝右前叶 right anterior lobe of liver

9　肝左内叶 left medial lobe of liver

10　肝左外叶 left lateral lobe of liver

11　肝尾状叶 caudate lobe of liver

12　胸主动脉 thoracic aorta

13　左膈脚 left crus of diaphragm

14　半奇静脉 hemiazygos vein

15　右膈脚 right crus of diaphragm

16　下腔静脉 inferior vena cava

17　肝门静脉右后支 posterior branch of right hepatic portal vein

18　肝门静脉右前支 anterior branch of right hepatic portal vein

19　网膜囊上隐窝 superior recess of omental bursa

20　肝门静脉左支囊部 sac part of left hepatic portal vein

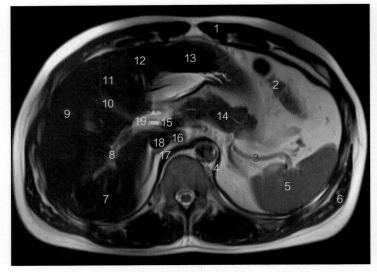

图 4-8　经肝门下方的横断层 MR T$_2$ 加权图像

1	腹直肌 rectus abdominis	2	横结肠 transverse colon
3	脾静脉 splenic vein	4	左膈脚 left crus of diaphragm
5	脾 spleen	6	背阔肌 latissimus dorsi
7	肝右后叶 right posterior lobe of liver		
8	肝门静脉右后下支 right posteroinferior branch of hepatic portal vein		
9	肝右前叶 right anterior lobe of liver	10	胆囊 gallbladder
11	肝左内叶 left medial lobe of liver	12	肝左外叶 left lateral lobe of liver
13	胃体 body of stomach	14	胰体 body of pancreas
15	门腔间隙 portacaval space	16	肝尾状叶 candate lobe of liver
17	右膈脚 right crus of diaphragm	18	下腔静脉 inferior vena cava
19	肝门静脉右支 right hepatic portal vein		

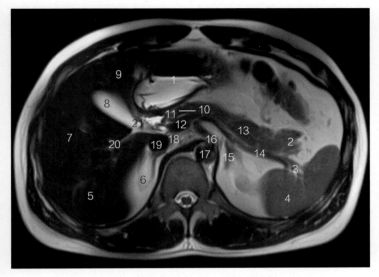

图 4-9　经腹腔干的横断层 MR T$_2$ 加权图像

1	胃体 body of stomach	2	胰尾 tail of pancreas
3	脾门 splenic hilum	4	脾 spleen
5	肝右后叶 right posterior lobe of liver		
6	右肾上腺三角 right suprarenal gland triangle		
7	肝右前叶 right anterior lobe of liver	8	胆囊 gallbladder
9	肝左内叶 left medial lobe of liver	10	胰颈 neck of pancreas
11	胰头 head of pancreas		
12	肠系膜上静脉 superior mesenteric vein		
13	胰体 body of pancreas	14	脾静脉 splenic vein
15	左肾上腺 left suprarenal gland	16	腹腔干 celiac trunk
17	腹主动脉 abdominal aorta	18	尾状突 caudate process
19	下腔静脉 inferior vena cava		
20	肝门右切迹 right notch of portal hepatis		
21	胆囊管 cystic duct		

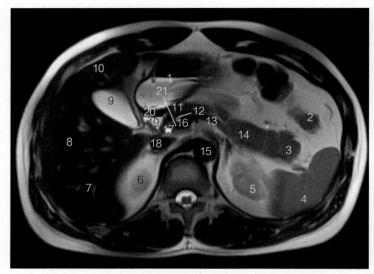

图 4-10 经肝门静脉合成处的横断层 MR T$_2$ 加权图像

1	胃体 body of stomach	2	结肠左曲 left colic flexure
3	胰尾 tail of pancreas	4	脾 spleen
5	左肾 left kidney	6	右肾 right kidney
7	肝右后叶 right posterior lobe of liver		
8	肝右前叶 right anterior lobe of liver		
9	胆囊 gallbladder	10	肝左内叶 left medial lobe of liver
11	胰颈 neck of pancreas	12	胰管 pancreatic duct
13	脾静脉 splenic vein	14	胰体 body of pancreas
15	腹主动脉 abdominal aorta		
16	肠系膜上静脉 superior mesenteric vein		
17	胆总管 common bile duct	18	下腔静脉 inferior vena cava
19	十二指肠上部 superior part of duodenum		
20	幽门 pylorus		
21	胰钩突 uncinate process of pancreas		

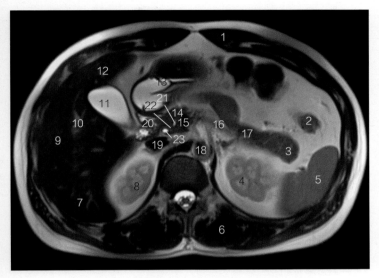

图 4-11 经胆囊体的横断层 MR T₂ 加权图像

1 腹直肌 rectus abdominis　　　　　2 结肠左曲 left colic flexure

3 胰尾 tail of pancreas　　　　　　4 左肾 left kidney

5 脾 spleen　　　　　　　　　　6 竖脊肌 erector spinae

7 肝右后叶 right posterior lobe of liver　　8 右肾 right kidney

9 肝右前叶 right anterior lobe of lvier

10 肝门静脉右前下支 right anteroinferior branch of hepatic portal vein

11 胆囊体 body of gallbladder　　　12 肝左内叶 left medial lobe of liver

13 胃体 body of stomach　　　　　14 胰颈 neck of pancreas

15 肠系膜上静脉 superior mesenteric vein

16 脾静脉 splenic vein　　　　　　17 胰体 body of pancreas

18 腹主动脉 abdominal aorta　　　　19 下腔静脉 inferior vena cava

20 十二指肠上部 superior part of duodenum

21 胰管 pancreatic duct　　　　　　22 钩突 uncinate process

23 胆总管 common bile duct

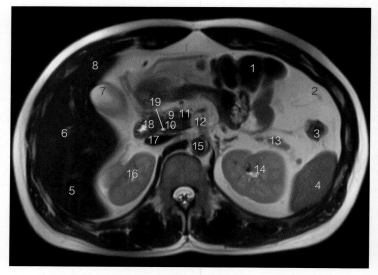

图 4-12   经胰头下份的横断层 MR T$_2$ 加权图像

1   横结肠 transverse colon   2   大网膜 greater omentum

3   降结肠 descending colon   4   脾 spleen

5   肝右后叶 right posterior lobe of liver

6   肝右前叶 right anterior lobe of liver   7   胆囊 gallbladder

8   肝左内叶 left medial lobe of liver   9   胰头 head of pancreas

10   胰管 pancreatic duct

11   肠系膜上静脉 superior mesenteric vein

12   肠系膜上动脉 superior mesenteric artery

13   胰体 body of pancreas   14   左肾 left kidney

15   腹主动脉 abdominal aorta   16   右肾 right kidney

17   下腔静脉 inferior vena cava

18   十二指肠降部 descending part of duodenum

19   胆总管 common bile duct

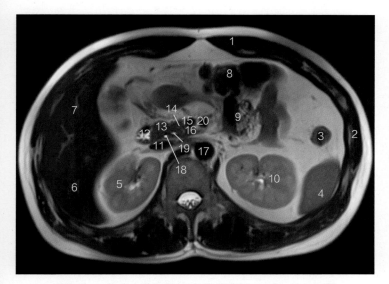

图 4-13 经十二指肠空肠曲的横断层 MR T$_2$加权图像

1	腹直肌 rectus abdominis	2	腹外侧肌肉 lateral abdominal muscle
3	降结肠 descending colon	4	脾 spleen
5	右肾 right kidney	6	肝右后叶 right posterior lobe of liver
7	肝右前叶 right anterior lobe of liver		
8	横结肠 transverse colon	9	十二指肠空肠曲 duodenojejunal flexure
10	左肾 left kidney	11	下腔静脉 inferior vena cava
12	十二指肠降部 descending part of duodenum		
13	十二指肠水平部 horizontal part of duodenum		
14	胰头 head of pancreas	15	肠系膜上静脉 superior mesenteric vein
16	胰钩突 uncinate process of pancreas		
17	腹主动脉 abdominal aorta	18	胆总管 common bile duct
19	胰管 pancreatic duct		
20	肠系膜上动脉 superior mesenteric artery		

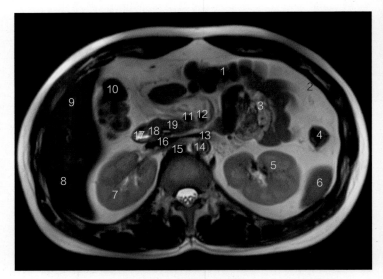

图 4-14　经十二指肠大乳头的横断层 MR T$_2$ 加权图像

1	横结肠 transverse colon	2	大网膜 greater omentum
3	空肠 jejunum	4	降结肠 descending colon
5	左肾 left kidney	6	脾 spleen
7	右肾 right kidney		
8	肝右后叶 right posterior lobe of liver		
9	肝右前叶 right anterior lobe of liver		
10	结肠右曲 right colic flexure		
11	肠系膜上静脉 superior mesenteric vein		
12	肠系膜上动脉 superior mesenteric artery		
13	左肾静脉 left renal vein	14	腹主动脉 abdominal aorta
15	右膈脚 right crus of diaphragm	16	下腔静脉 inferior vena cava
17	十二指肠降部 descending part of duodenum		
18	十二指肠大乳头 major duodenal papilla		
19	十二指肠水平部 horizontal part of duodenum		

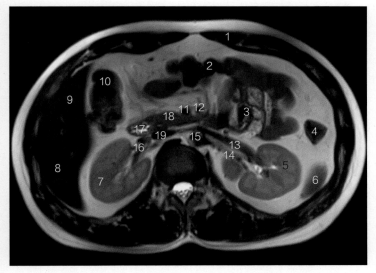

图 4-15　经肾门上份的横断层 MR T$_2$ 加权图像

1	腹直肌 rectus abdominis	2	横结肠 transverse colon
3	空肠 jejunum	4	降结肠 descending colon
5	左肾 left kidney	6	脾 spleen

7　右肾 right kidney

8　肝右后叶 right posterior lobe of liver

9　肝右前叶 right anterior lobe of liver

10　升结肠 ascending colon

11　肠系膜上静脉 superior mesenteric vein

12　肠系膜上动脉 superior mesenteric artery

13	左肾静脉 left renal vein	14	左肾动脉 left renal artery
15	腹主动脉 abdominal aorta	16	右肾静脉 right renal vein

17　十二指肠降部 descending part of duodenum

18　十二指肠水平部 horizontal part of duodenum

19　下腔静脉 inferior vena cava

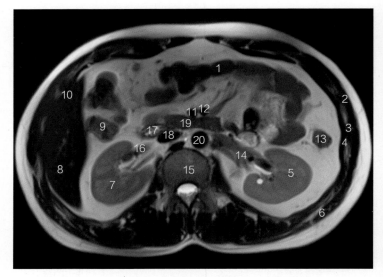

图 4-16 经肾门中份的横断层 MR T$_2$ 加权图像

1 横结肠 transverse colon   2 腹外斜肌 obliquus externus abdominis

3 腹内斜肌 obliquus internus abdominis

4 腹横肌 transversus abdominis

5 左肾 left kidney   6 背阔肌 latissimus dorsi

7 右肾 right kidney   8 肝右后叶 right posterior lobe of liver

9 升结肠 ascending colon   10 肝右前叶 right anterior lobe of liver

11 肠系膜上静脉 superior mesenteric vein

12 肠系膜上动脉 superior mesenteric artery

13 降结肠 descending colon   14 左肾静脉 left renal vein

15 第 2 腰椎椎体 body of 2nd lumbar vertebrae

16 右肾静脉 right renal vein   17 十二指肠降部 descending part of duodenum

18 下腔静脉 inferior vena cava

19 十二指肠水平部 horizontal part of duodenum

20 腹主动脉 abdominal aorta

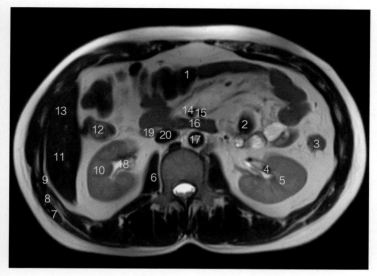

图 4-17　经肾门下份的横断层 MR T₂ 加权图像

1 　横结肠 transverse colon	2 　空肠 jejunum
3 　降结肠 descending colon	4 　左肾门 left renal hilum
5 　左肾 left kidney	6 　腰大肌 psoas major
7 　腹外斜肌 obliquus externus abdominis	
8 　腹内斜肌 obliquus internus abdominis	
9 　腹横肌 transversus abdominis	10 　右肾 right kidney
11 　肝右后叶 right posterior lobe of liver	12 　升结肠 ascending colon
13 　肝右前叶 right anterior lobe of liver	
14 　肠系膜上静脉 superior mesenteric vein	
15 　肠系膜上动脉 superior mesenteric artery	
16 　十二指肠水平部 horizontal part of duodenum	
17 　腹主动脉 abdominal aorta	18 　右肾门 right renal hilum
19 　十二指肠降部 descending part of duodenum	
20 　下腔静脉 inferior vena cava	

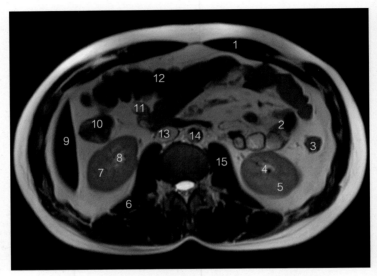

图 4-18 经左右肾窦的横断层 MR T₂ 加权图像

1 腹直肌 rectus abdominis	2 空肠 jejunum
3 降结肠 descending colon	4 左肾窦 left renal sinus
5 左肾 left kidney	6 腰方肌 quadratus lumborum
7 右肾 right kidney	8 右肾窦 right renal sinus
9 肝右叶 right lobe of liver	10 升结肠 ascending colon
11 回肠 ileum	12 横结肠 transverse colon
13 下腔静脉 inferior vena cava	14 腹主动脉 abdominal aorta
15 腰大肌 psoas major	

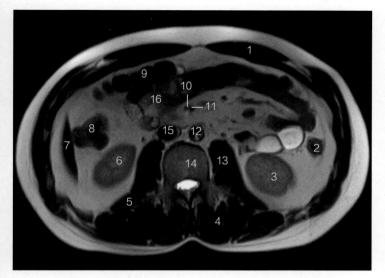

图 4-19　经第 3 腰椎椎体的横断层 MR T₂ 加权图像

1　腹直肌 rectus abdominis
2　降结肠 descending colon
3　左肾 left kidney
4　竖脊肌 erector spinae
5　腰方肌 quadratus lumborum
6　右肾 right kidney
7　肝右叶 right lobe of liver
8　升结肠 ascending colon
9　横结肠 transverse colon
10　肠系膜上静脉 superior mesenteric vein
11　肠系膜上动脉 superior mesenteric artery
12　腹主动脉 abdominal aorta
13　腰大肌 psoas major
14　第 3 腰椎椎体 body of 3rd lumbar vertebrae
15　下腔静脉 inferior vena cava
16　回肠 ileum

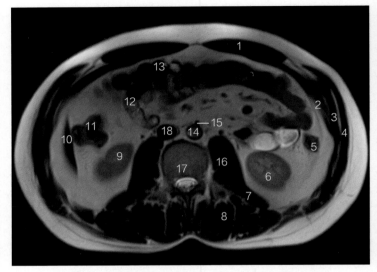

图 4-20　经肠系膜下动脉的横断层 MR T$_2$ 加权图像

1	腹直肌 rectus abdominis	2	腹横肌 transversus abdominis

3　腹内斜肌 obliquus internus abdominis

4　腹外斜肌 obliquus externus abdominis

5	降结肠 descending colon	6	左肾 left kidney
7	腰方肌 quadratus lumborum	8	竖脊肌 erector spinae
9	右肾 right kidney	10	肝右叶 right lobe of liver
11	升结肠 ascending colon	12	回肠 ileum
13	横结肠 transverse colon	14	腹主动脉 abdominal aorta

15　肠系膜下动脉 inferior mesenteric artery

16　腰大肌 psoas major

17　第 3 腰椎椎体 body of 3rd lumbar vertebrae

18　下腔静脉 inferior vena cava

第五章 腹部矢状断层 MR 图像

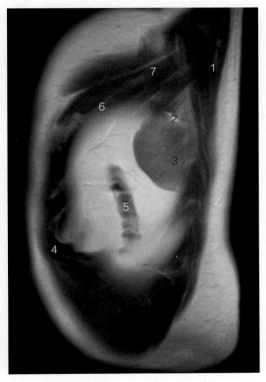

图 5-1　经降结肠的矢状断层 MR T$_2$ 加权图像

1　背阔肌 latissimus dorsi	2　肋膈隐窝 costodiaphragmatic recess
3　脾 spleen	4　腹外斜肌 obliquus externus abdominis
5　降结肠 descending colon	6　膈 diaphragm
7　左肺下叶 inferior lobe of left lung	

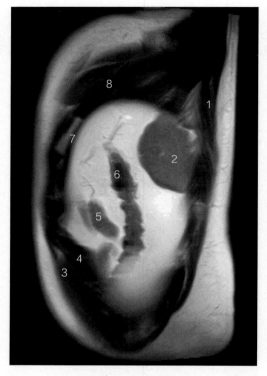

图 5-2　经回肠的矢状断层 MR T$_2$ 加权图像

1	背阔肌 latissimus dorsi	2	脾 spleen
3	腹外斜肌 obliquus externus abdominis	4	腹横肌 transversus abdominis
5	回肠 ileum	6	降结肠 descending colon
7	膈 diaphragm	8	左肺下叶 inferior lobe of left lung

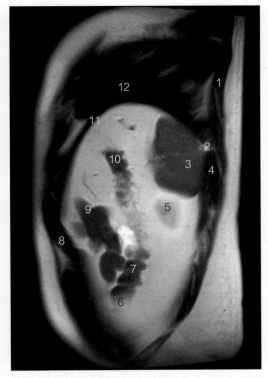

图 5-3 经结肠左曲的矢状断层 MR T$_2$ 加权图像

1 背阔肌 latissimus dorsi	2 肋膈隐窝 costodiaphragmatic recesses
3 脾 spleen	4 下后锯肌 serratus posterior inferior
5 左肾 left kidney	6 乙状结肠 sigmoid colon
7 降结肠 descending colon	8 腹横肌 transversus abdomimis
9 回肠 ileum	10 结肠左曲 left colic flexure
11 膈 diaphragm	12 左肺下叶 inferior lobe of left lung

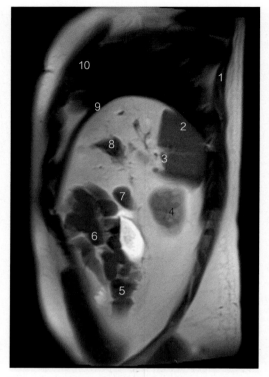

图 5-4 经左肾外侧的矢状断层 MR T₂ 加权图像

1	背阔肌 latissimus dorsi	2	脾 spleen
3	脾静脉 splenic vein	4	左肾 left kidney
5	乙状结肠 sigmoid colon	6	回肠 ileum
7	降结肠 descending colon	8	结肠左曲 left colic flexure
9	膈 diaphragm	10	左肺上叶 superior lobe of left lung

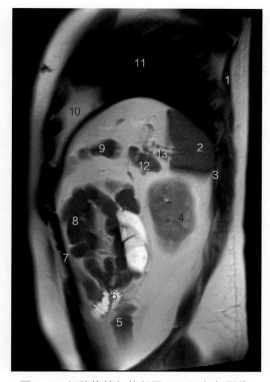

图 5-5 经胰体的矢状断层 MR T$_2$ 加权图像

1	背阔肌 latissimus dorsi	2	脾 spleen
3	膈 diaphragm	4	左肾 left kidney
5	乙状结肠 sigmoid colon	6	空肠 jejunum
7	腹横肌 transversus abdomimis	8	回肠 ileum
9	横结肠 transverse colon	10	心包外脂肪 pericadiac fat
11	左肺下叶 inferior lobe of left lung	12	胰体 body of pancreas
13	脾静脉 splenic vein		

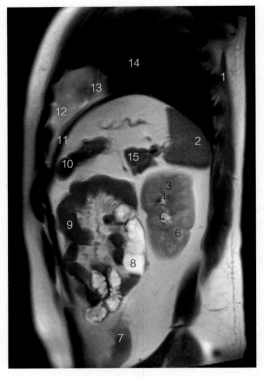

图 5-6　经脾门的矢状断层 MR T₂ 加权图像

1	背阔肌 latissimus dorsi	2	脾 spleen
3	左肾 left kidney	4	肾小盏 minor renal calice
5	左肾静脉 left renal vein	6	肾锥体 renal pyramid
7	乙状结肠 sigmoid colon	8	空肠 jejunum
9	回肠 ileum	10	横结肠 transverse colon
11	膈 diaphragm	12	心包外脂肪 pericadiac fat
13	心 heart		
14	左肺下叶 inferior lobe of left lung	15	胰体 body of pancreas

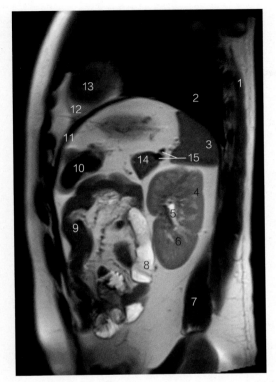

图 5-7　经左肾门左侧份的矢状断层 MR T$_2$ 加权图像

1	竖脊肌 erector spinae	2	左肺下叶 inferior lobe of left lung
3	脾 spleen	4	左肾 left kidney
5	肾大盏 major renal calice	6	肾锥体 renal pyramid
7	腰方肌 quadratus lumborum	8	空肠 jejunum
9	回肠 ileum	10	横结肠 transverse colon
11	膈 diaphragm	12	心包外脂肪 pericardiac fat
13	左心室 left ventricle	14	胰体 body of pancreas
15	脾动、静脉 splenic artery and vein		

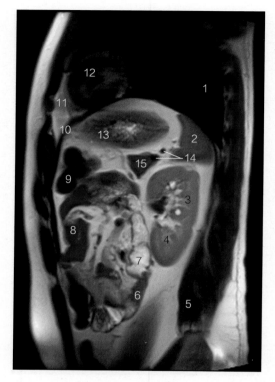

图 5-8　经左肾门中份的矢状断层 MR T$_2$ 加权图像

1　左肺下叶 inferior lobe of left lung	2　脾 spleen
3　左肾 left kidney	4　肾锥体 renal pyramid
5　腰方肌 quadratus lumborum	6　乙状结肠 sigmoid colon
7　空肠 jejunum	8　回肠 ileum
9　横结肠 transverse colon	10　膈 diaphragm
11　心包外脂肪 pericadiac fat	12　左心室 left ventricle
13　胃底 fundus of stomach	
14　脾动、静脉 splenic artery and vein	15　胰体 body of pancreas

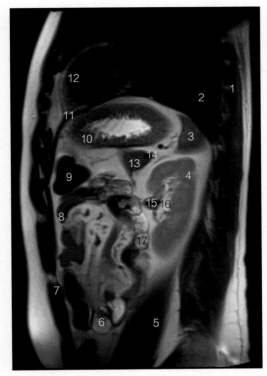

图 5-9 经左肾门右侧份的矢状断层 MR T₂ 加权图像

1	竖脊肌 erector spinae	2	左肺下叶 inferior lobe of left lung
3	脾 spleen	4	左肾 left kidney
5	腰大肌 psoas major	6	乙状结肠 sigmoid colon
7	腹直肌 rectus abdominis	8	回肠 ileum
9	横结肠 transverse colon	10	胃底 fundus of stomach
11	膈 diaphragm	12	左心室 left ventricle
13	胰体 body of pancreas	14	脾静脉 splenic vein
15	肾动、静脉 renal artery and vein	16	肾盂 renal pelvis
17	空肠 jejunum		

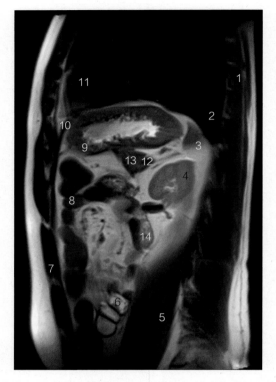

图 5-10　经脾前端的矢状断层 MR T₂ 加权图像

1　竖脊肌 erector spinae	2　左肺下叶 inferior lobe of left lung
3　脾 spleen	4　左肾 left kidney
5　腰大肌 psoas major	6　乙状结肠 sigmoid colon
7　腹直肌 rectus abdominis	8　回肠 ileum
9　胃底 fundus of stomach	10　膈 diaphragm
11　左心室 left ventricle	12　脾动脉 splenic artery
13　胰体 body of pancreas	14　空肠 jejumum

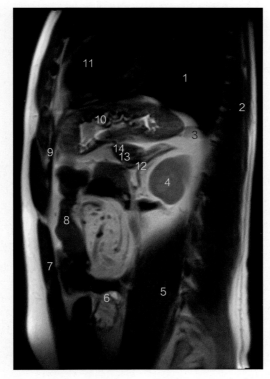

图 5-11　经左肾内侧的矢状断层 MR T$_2$ 加权图像

1　左肺下叶 inferior lobe of left lung	2　竖脊肌 erector spinae
3　脾 spleen	4　左肾 left kidney
5　腰大肌 psoas major	6　乙状结肠 sigmoid colon
7　腹直肌 erector abdominis	8　回肠 ileum
9　膈 diaphragm	10　胃体 body of stomach
11　右心室 right ventricle	12　左肾上腺 left suprarenal gland
13　胰体 body of pancreas	14　主胰管 main pancreatic duct

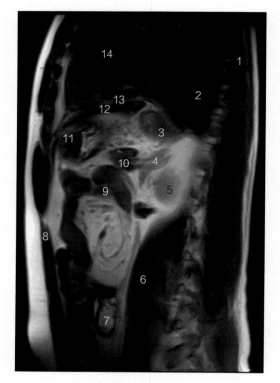

图 5-12   经肝左上角的矢状断层 MR T₂ 加权图像

1　竖脊肌 erector spinae	2　左肺下叶 inferior lobe of left lung
3　脾 spleen	4　左肾上腺 left supralrenal gland
5　左肾 left kidney	6　腰大肌 psoas major
7　乙状结肠 sigmoid colon	8　腹直肌 rectus abdominis
9　回肠 ileum	10　胰体 body of pancreas
11　胃体 body of stomach	12　肝左外叶 left lateral lobe of liver
13　膈 diaphragm	14　右心室 right ventricle

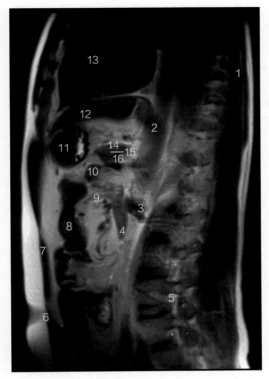

图 5-13 经网膜囊的矢状断层 MR T₂ 加权图像

1	竖脊肌 erector spinae	2	膈 diaphragm
3	肾动脉 renal artery		
4	十二指肠升部 ascending part of duodenum		
5	腰神经 lumbar nerve	6	白线 white line
7	腹直肌 rectus abdominis	8	回肠 ileum
9	网膜囊 omental bursa	10	横结肠 transverse colon
11	胃体 body of stomach		
12	肝左外叶 left lateral lobe of liver	13	右心室 right ventricle
14	主胰管 main pancreatic duct	15	胰体 body of pancreas
16	脾动脉 splenic artery		

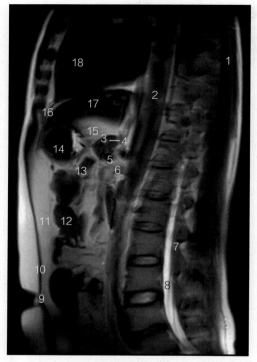

图 5-14 经脐的矢状断层 MR T$_2$ 加权图像

1　竖脊肌 erector spinae　　　　2　胸主动脉 thoracic aorta

3　主胰管 main pancreatic duct　　4　胰体 body of pancreas

5　脾静脉 splenic vein

6　肠系膜上动脉 superior mesenteric artery

7　棘间韧带 interspinal ligament

8　马尾 cauda equina　　　　　　9　脐 umbilical region

10　白线 white line　　　　　　　11　大网膜 greater omentum

12　回肠 ileum　　　　　　　　　13　横结肠 transverse colon

14　胃体 body of stomach　　　　 15　小网膜 lesser omentum

16　膈 diaphragm　　　　　　　　17　肝左外叶 left lateral lobe of liver

18　右心室 right ventricle

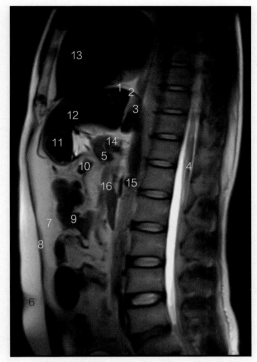

图 5-15　经胰颈的矢状断层 MR T$_2$ 加权图像

1	肝裸区 bare area of liver	2	膈 diaphragm
3	肝尾状叶 caudate lobe of liver	4	马尾 cauda equina
5	脾静脉 splenic vein	6	脐 umbilical region
7	大网膜 great omentum	8	白线 white line
9	回肠 ileum	10	横结肠 transverse colon
11	胃体 body of stomach	12	肝左外叶 left lateral lobe of liver
13	右心室 right ventricle	14	胰颈 neck of pancreas
15	左肾动脉 left renal artery		
16	十二指肠水平部 horizontal part of duodenum		

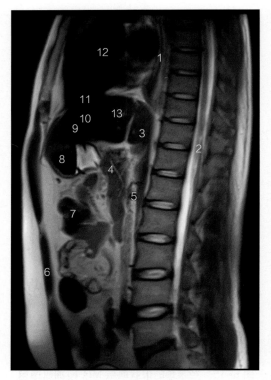

图 5-16　经肝门静脉左外上支和左外下支的矢状断层 MR T$_2$ 加权图像

1 食管 esophagus	2 马尾 cauda equina
3 肝尾状叶 caudate lobe of liver	4 胰头 head of pancreas
5 右肾动脉 right renal artery	6 腹直肌 rectus abdominis
7 空肠 jejunum	8 胃体 body of stomach

9　肝门静脉左外下支 left lateroinferior branch of hepatic portal vein

10　肝左外叶 left lateral lobe of liver	11　膈 diaphragm
12　右心室 right ventricle	

13　肝门静脉左外上支 left laterosuperior branch of hepatic vein

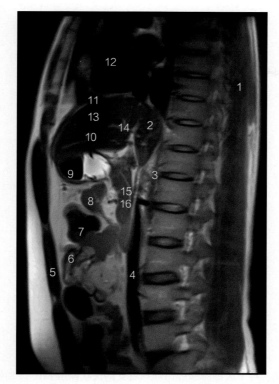

图 5-17 经十二指肠空肠曲的矢状断层 MR T₂ 加权图像

1　竖脊肌 erector spinae　　　　　2　肝尾状叶 caudate lobe of liver

3　右膈脚 right crus of disphragm

4　下腔静脉 inferior vena cava　5　腹直肌 rectus abdominis

6　回肠 ileum　　　　　　　　　　7　空肠 jejunum

8　十二指肠空肠曲 duodenojejunal flexure

9　胃体 body of stomach　　　　10　肝门静脉左支 left hepatic portal vein

11　膈 diaphragm　　　　　　　12　右心室 right ventricle

13　肝左外叶 left lateral lobe of liver

14　肝门静脉右支 right hepatic portal vein

15　胰头 head of pancreas　　　16　主胰管 main pancreatic duct

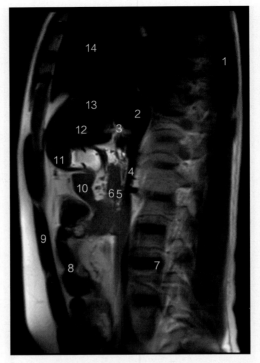

图 5-18　经下腔静脉和肝门静脉右支的矢状断层 MR T$_2$ 加权图像

1　竖脊肌 erector spinae	2　肝尾状叶 caudate lobe of liver
3　肝门静脉右支 right hepatic portal vein	
4　下腔静脉 inferior vena cava	5　胰管 pancreatic duct
6　胰 pancreas	7　椎间盘 intervertebral disc
8　空肠 jejunum	9　腹直肌 rectus abdominis
10　横结肠 transverse colon	11　胃窦部 antrum of stomach
12　肝门静脉左支 left hepatic portal vein	
13　肝左叶 left lobe of liver	14　右肺中叶 middle lobe of right lung

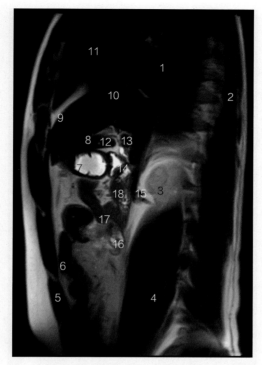

图 5-19 经十二指肠球部的矢状断层 MR T₂ 加权图像

1　右肺下叶 inferior lobe of right lung　　2　竖脊肌 erector spinae

3　右肾 right kidney　　　　　　　　　　4　腰大肌 psoas major

5　腹直肌 rectus abdominis　　　　　　　6　回肠 ileum

7　胃幽门部 pyloric part of stomach

8　肝门静脉左支 left hepatic portal vein

9　膈 diaphragm　　　　　　　　　　　10　肝左叶 left lobe of liver

11　右肺中叶 middle lobe of right lung　　12　肝左内叶 left medial lobe of liver

13　肝门静脉右支 right hepatic portal vein

14　十二指肠上部 superior part of duodenum

15　右肾动脉 right renal artery　　　　　16　空肠 jejunum

17　横结肠 transverse colon　　　　　　18　胰头 head of pancreas

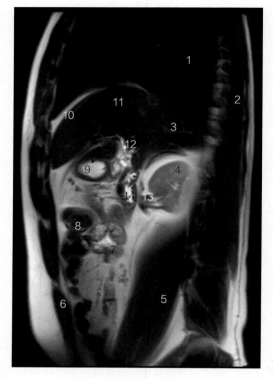

图 5-20 经右肾内侧份的矢状断层 MR T$_2$ 加权图像

1 右肺下叶 inferior lobe of right lung

2 竖脊肌 erector spinae

3 肝右后叶 right posterior lobe of liver

4 右肾 right kidney

5 腰大肌 psoas major

6 腹直肌 rectus abdominis

7 回肠 ileum

8 横结肠 transverse colon

9 胃幽门部 pyloric part of stomach

10 膈 diaphragm

11 肝右前叶 right anterior lobe of liver

12 肝门静脉 hepatic portal vein

13 右肾动脉 right renal artery

14 十二指肠降部 descending part of duodenum

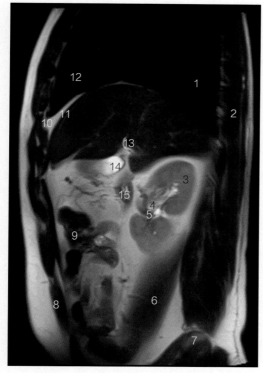

图 5-21　经右肾窦的矢状断层 MR T₂ 加权图像

1　右肺下叶 inferior lobe of right lung
2　竖脊肌 erector spinae
3　右肾 right kidney
4　右肾窦 right renal sinus
5　肾动、静脉 renal artery and vein
6　腰大肌 psoas major
7　髂骨 ilium
8　腹直肌 rectus abdominis
9　回肠 ileum
10　胸膜腔 pleural cavity
11　膈 diaphragm
12　右肺中叶 middle lobe of left lung
13　肝门静脉右支 right hepatic portal vein
14　胆囊颈 neck of gallbladder
15　十二指肠 duodenum

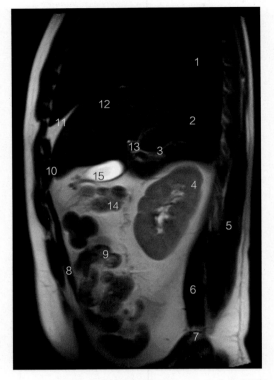

图 5-22 经结肠右曲的矢状断层 MR T₂ 加权图像

1 右肺下叶 inferior lobe of right lung

2 肝右后叶 right posterior lobe of liver

3 肝门静脉右后下支 right posteroinferior branch of hepatic portal vein

4 右肾 right kidney   5 竖脊肌 erector spinae

6 腰方肌 quadratus lumborum   7 髂骨翼 ilium

8 腹直肌 rectus abdominis   9 回肠 ileum

10 膈 diaphragm   11 胸膜腔 pleural cavity

12 肝右前叶 right anterior lobe of liver

13 肝门静脉右前支 right anterior branch of hepatic portal vein

14 结肠右曲 right colic flexure   15 胆囊 gallbladder

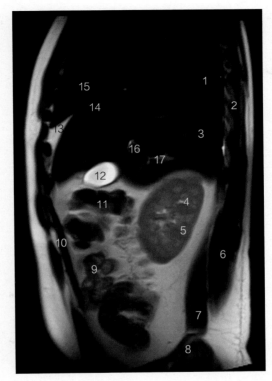

图 5-23 经肝门静脉右支的矢状断层 MR T$_2$ 加权图像

1	右肺下叶 inferior lobe of right lung	2	背阔肌 latisimus dorsi
3	肝右后叶 right posterior lobe of liver	4	右肾 right kidney
5	肾锥体 renal pyramid	6	竖脊肌 erector spinae
7	腰方肌 quadratus lumborum	8	髂骨翼 ilium
9	回肠 ileum	10	腹横肌 transversus abdominis
11	结肠右曲 right colic flexure	12	胆囊体 body of gallbladder
13	胸膜腔 pleural cavity	14	肝右前叶 right anterior lobe of liver
15	右肺中叶 middle lobe of right lung		

16　肝门静脉右前支 right anterior branch of hepatic portal vein

17　肝门静脉右后支 right posterior branch of hepatic portal vein

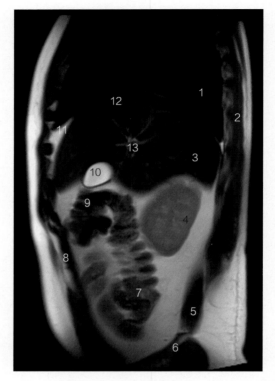

图 5-24 经右肾外侧份和胆囊的矢状断层 MR T₂ 加权图像

1 右肺下叶 inferior lobe of right lung	2 竖脊肌 erector spinae
3 肝右后叶 right posterior lobe of liver	4 右肾 right kidney
5 腰方肌 quadratus lumborum	6 髂骨翼 ilium
7 升结肠 ascending colon	
8 腹横肌 transversus abdominis	9 回肠 ileum
10 胆囊体 body of gallbladder	11 胸膜腔 pleural cavity
12 肝右前叶 right anterior lobe of liver	
13 肝门静脉右前支 right anterior branch of hepatic portal vein	

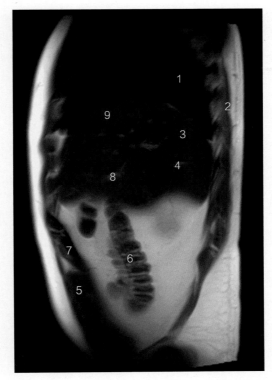

图 5-25　经升结肠的矢状断层 MR T$_2$ 加权图像

1　右肺下叶 infeirior lobe of right lung

2　背阔肌 latissimus dorsi

3　肝右后叶 right posterior lobe of liver

4　肝门静脉右后下支 right posteroinferior branch of hepatic portal vein

5　腹内斜肌 obliquus internus abdominis

6　升结肠 ascending colon

7　腹横肌 transversus abdominis

8　肝门静脉右前下支 right anteroinferior branch of hepatic portal vein

9　肝右前叶 right anterior lobe of liver

第六章　腹部冠状断层 MR 图像

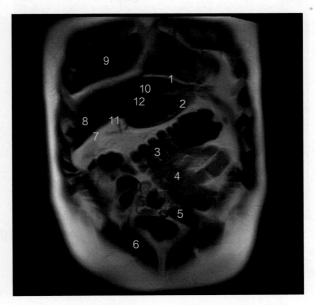

图 6-1　经肝圆韧带的冠状断层 MR T$_2$ 加权图像

1　膈 diaphragm

3　横结肠 transverse colon

5　回肠 ileum

7　右肝下间隙 right subhepatic space

9　右肺中叶 middle lobe of right lung

11　肝圆韧带 ligamentum teres hepatis

2　胃体 body of stomach

4　空肠 jejunum

6　腹直肌 rectus abdominis

8　肝左内叶 left medial lobe of liver

10　肝左外叶 left lateral lobe of liver

12　肝门静脉左外上支 left superolateral branch of hepatic portal vein

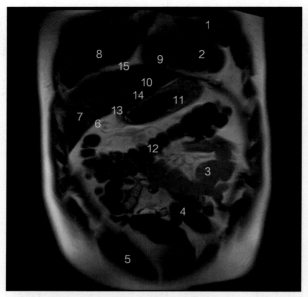

图 6-2　经肝圆韧带和肝门静脉左外下支的冠状断层 MR T$_2$ 加权图像

1　左肺上叶 superior lobe of left lung	2　左心室 left ventricle
3　空肠 jejunum	4　回肠 ileum
5　腹直肌 rectus abdominis	6　右肝下间隙 right subhepatic space
7　肝左内叶 left medial lobe of liver	8　右肺中叶 middle lobe of right lung
9　右心室 right ventricle	10　肝左外叶 left lateral lobe of liver
11　胃体 body of stomach	12　横结肠 transverse colon

13　肝圆韧带 ligamentum teres hepatis

14　肝门静脉左外下支 left lateroinferior branch of hepatic portal vein

15　肝裸区 bare area of liver

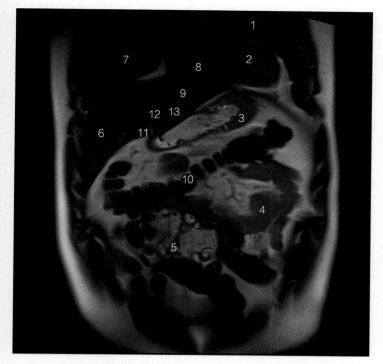

图 6-3　经肝左静脉属支和肝门静脉左外下支的冠状断层 MR T₂ 加权图像

1 　左肺上叶 superior lobe of left lung
2 　左心室 left ventricle
3 　胃体 body of stomach
4 　空肠 jejunum
5 　回肠 ileum
6 　肝右前叶 right anterior lobe of liver
7 　右肺中叶 middle lobe of right lung
8 　右心室 right ventricle
9 　肝左外叶 left lateral lobe of liver
10 　横结肠 transverse colon
11 　肝圆韧带 ligamentum teres hepatis
12 　肝门静脉左外下支 left lateroinferior branch of hepatic portal vein
13 　肝左静脉属支 tributaries of left hepatic vein

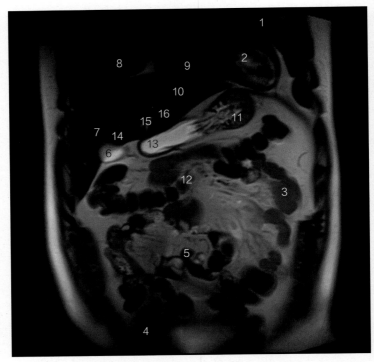

图 6-4　经胆囊体和肝门静脉左支囊部的冠状断层 MR T$_2$ 加权图像

1　左肺上叶 superior lobe of left lung

2　左心室 left ventricle

3　空肠 jejunum

4　腹直肌 rectus abdominis

5　回肠 ileum

6　胆囊体 body of gallbladder

7　肝右前叶 right anterior lobe of liver

8　右肺中叶 middle lobe of right lung

9　右心室 right ventricle

10　肝左外叶 left lateral lobe of liver

11　胃体 body of stomach

12　横结肠 transverse colon

13　十二指肠上部 superior part of duodenum

14　肝门静脉右前下支 right anteroinferior branch of hepatic portal vein

15　肝左静脉左支囊部 sac part of left hepatic portal vein

16　肝门静脉左外下支 left lateroinferior branch of hepatic portal vein

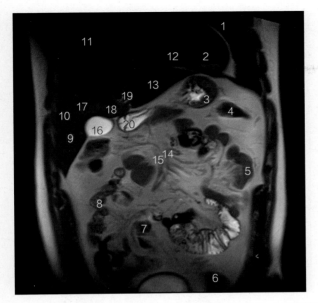

图 6-5 经肝门静脉左支矢状部的冠状断层 MR T₂ 加权图像

1 左肺上叶 superior lobe of left lung
2 左心室 left ventricle
3 胃体 body of stomach
4 横结肠 transverse colon
5 空肠 jejunum
6 腹直肌 rectus abdominis
7 回肠 ileum
8 升结肠 ascending colon
9 肝右静脉右前下支 right anteroinferior branch of hepatic portal vein
10 肝右前叶 right anterior lobe of liver
11 右肺中叶 middle lobe of right lung
12 右心室 right ventricle
13 肝左外叶 left lateral lobe of liver
14 肠系膜上动脉 superior mesenteric artery
15 肠系膜上静脉 superior mesenteric vein
16 胆囊体 body of gallbladder
17 肝中静脉属支 tributaries of middle hepatic vein
18 肝左内叶 left medial lobe of liver
19 肝门静脉左支矢状部 sagittal part of left hepatic portal vein
20 十二指肠上部 superior part of duodenum

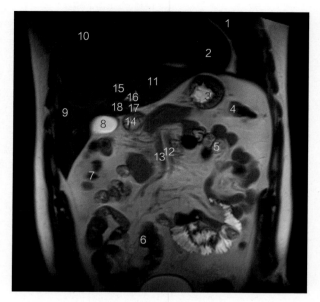

图 6-6 经肝门静脉左支角部的冠状断层 MR T$_2$加权图像

1 左肺上叶 superior lobe of left lung
2 左心室 left ventricle
3 胃体 body of stomach
4 横结肠 transverse colon
5 空肠 jejunum
6 回肠 ileum
7 升结肠 ascending colon
8 胆囊体 body of gallbladder
9 肝右前叶 right anterior lobe of liver
10 右肺中叶 middle lobe of right lung
11 肝左外叶 left lateral lobe of liver
12 肠系膜上动脉 superior mesenteric artery
13 肠系膜上静脉 superior mesenteric vein
14 十二指肠上部 superior part of duodenum
15 肝中静脉属支 tributaries of middle hepatic vein
16 肝门静脉左支角部 angular part of left hepatic portal vein
17 肝圆韧带裂 fissure for ligamentum teres hepatis
18 肝左内叶 left medial lobe of liver

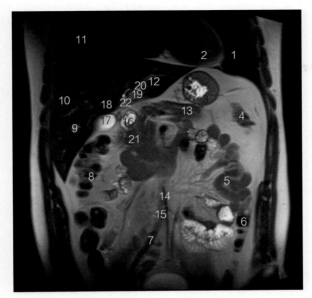

图 6-7　经肝门静脉左支横部的冠状断层 MR T$_2$ 加权图像

1	左肺下叶 inferior lobe of left lung	2	左心室 left ventricle
3	胃体 body of stomach	4	结肠左曲 left colic flexure
5	空肠 jejunum	6	降结肠 descending colon
7	右髂总动脉 right common iliac artery	8	升结肠 ascending colon
9	肝门静脉右前下支 right anteroinferior branch of hepatic portal vein		
10	肝右前叶 right anterior lobe of liver		
11	右肺中叶 middle lobe of right lung	12	肝左外叶 left lateral lobe of liver
13	胰体 body of pancreas		
14	肠系膜下动脉 inferior mesenteric artery		
15	腹主动脉 abdominal aorta		
16	十二指肠上部 superior part of duodenum		
17	胆囊体 body of gallbladder	18	肝左内叶 left medial lobe of liver
19	肝门静脉左支横部 transverse part of left hepatic portal vein		
20	肝门静脉左外上支 left laterosuperior branch of hepatic portal vein		
21	胰头 head of pancreas	22	小网膜 lesser omentum

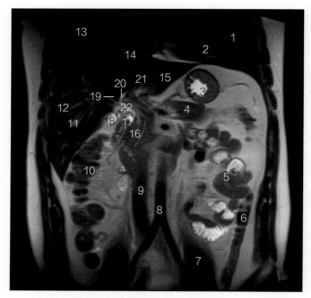

图 6-8　经肝门静脉主干的冠状断层 MR T₂ 加权图像

1　左肺下叶 inferior lobe of left lung　　　2　左心室 left ventricle

3　胃体 body of stomach　　　4　胰体 body of pancreas

5　空肠 jejunum　　　6　降结肠 descending colon

7　腰大肌 psoas major　　　8　腹主动脉 abdominal aorta

9　下腔静脉 inferior vena cava　　　10　升结肠 ascending colon

11　肝门静脉右前下支 right anteroinferior branch of hepatic portal vein

12　肝右前叶 right anterior lobe of liver

13　右肺下叶 inferior lobe of right lung　　　14　肝裸区 bare area of liver

15　肝左外叶 left lateral lobe of liver　　　16　胰头 head of pancreas

17　十二指肠降部 descending part of duodenum

18　胆囊体 body of gallbladder　　　19　肝左内叶 left medial lobe of liver

20　肝门静脉左支横部 transverse part of left hepatic portal vein

21　肝门静脉左外上支 left laterosuperior branch of hepatic portal vein

22　肝门静脉主干 trunk of hepatic portal vein

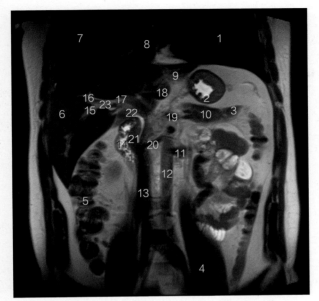

图 6-9 经肝门的冠状断层 MR T₂ 加权图像

1 左肺下叶 inferior lobe of left lung	2 胃体 body of stomach
3 胰尾 tail of pancreas	4 腰大肌 psoas major
5 升结肠 ascending colon	6 肝右前叶 right anterior lobe of liver
7 右肺下叶 inferior lobe of right lung	8 右心房 right atrium
9 肝左外叶 left lateral lobe of liver	10 胰体 body of pancreas
11 左肾动脉 left renal artery	12 腹主动脉 abdominal aorta

13 下腔静脉 inferior vena cava

14 十二指肠降部 descending part of duodenum

15 肝门静脉右后下支 right posteroinferior branch of hepatic portal vein

16 肝门静脉右后上支 right posterosuperior branch of hepatic portal vein

17 肝门静脉左支横部 transverse part of left hepatic portal vein

18 肝尾状叶 caudate lobe of liver	19 脾动脉 splenic artery
20 右肾动脉 right renal artery	21 胰头 head of pancreas

22 肝门静脉主干 trunk of hepatic portal vein

23 肝门静脉右支 right hepatic portal vein

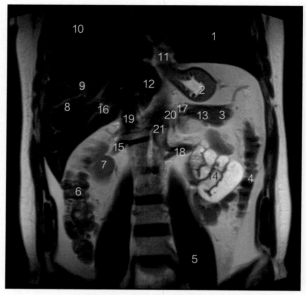

图 6–10　经食管腹段的冠状断层 MR T$_2$ 加权图像

1　左肺下叶 inferior lobe of left lung

2　胃体 body of stomach

3　胰尾 tail of pancreas

4　降结肠 descending colon

5　腰大肌 psoas major

6　升结肠 ascending colon

7　右肾 right kidney

8　肝右后叶 right posterior lobe of liver

9　肝门静脉右后上支 right posterosuperior branch of hepatic portal vein

10　右肺下叶 inferior lobe of right lung

11　食管腹段 abdominal part of esophagus

12　肝尾状叶 caudate lobe of liver

13　胰体 body of pancreas

14　空肠 jejunum

15　右肾静脉 right renal vein

16　肝门静脉右后下支 right posteroinferior branch of hepatic portal vein

17　脾动脉 splenic artery

18　左肾动脉 left renal artery

19　下腔静脉 inferior vena cava

20　腹腔干 celiac trunk

21　腹主动脉 abdominal aorta

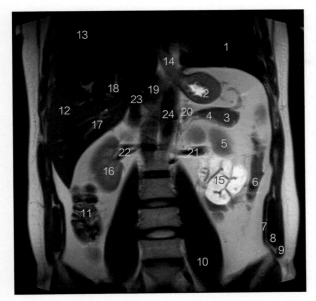

图 6-11　经下腔静脉后份和肝右静脉的冠状断层 MR T$_2$ 加权图像

1　左肺下叶 inferior lobe of left lung	2　胃体 body of stomach
3　胰尾 tail of pancreas	4　胰体 body of pancreas
5　左肾 left kidney	6　降结肠 descending colon
7　腹横肌 transversus abdominis	
8　腹内斜肌 obliquus internus abdominis	
9　腹外斜肌 obliquus externus abdominis	
10　腰大肌 psoas major	11　升结肠 ascending colon
12　肝右后叶 right posterior lobe of liver	13　右肺下叶 inferior lobe of right lung
14　食管 esophagus	15　空肠 jejunum
16　右肾 right kidney	
17　肝门静脉右后下支 right posteroinferior branch of hepatic portal vein	
18　肝右静脉 right hepatic vein	19　肝尾状叶 caudate lobe of liver
20　脾动脉 splenic artery	21　左肾动脉 left renal artery
22　右肾动脉 right renal artery	23　下腔静脉 inferior vena cava
24　腹主动脉 abdominal aorta	

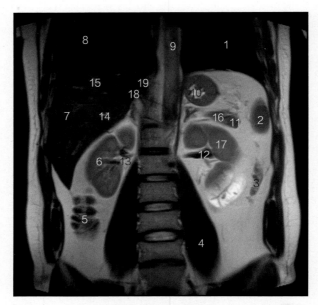

图6-12　经左、右肾门前份的冠状断层 MR T₂ 加权图像

1 左肺下叶 inferior lobe of left lung	2 脾 spleen
3 降结肠 descending colon	4 腰大肌 psoas major
5 升结肠 ascending colon	6 右肾 right kidney
7 肝右后叶 right posterior lobe of liver	8 右肺下叶 inferior lobe of right lung
9 腹主动脉 abdominal aorta	10 胃体 body of stomach
11 胰尾 tail of pancreas	12 左肾动脉 left renal artery

13 右肾门 right renal hilum

14 肝门静脉右后下支 right posteroinferior branch of hepatic portal vein

15 肝右静脉属支 tributaries of right hepatic vein

16 胰体 body of pancreas	17 左肾 left kidney
18 下腔静脉 inferior vena cava	19 肝尾状叶 caudate lobe of liver

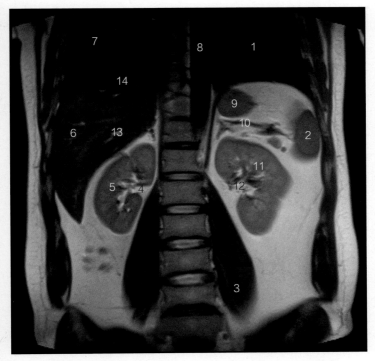

图 6-13 经左、右肾门中份的冠状断层 MR T₂ 加权图像

1 左肺下叶 inferior lobe of left lung	2 脾 spleen
3 腰大肌 psoas major	4 右肾门 right renal hilum
5 右肾 right kidney	6 肝右后叶 right posterior lobe of liver
7 右肺下叶 inferior lobe of right lung	8 腹主动脉 abdominal aorta
9 胃底 fundus of stomach	10 脾动脉 splenic artery
11 左肾 left kidney	12 左肾门 left renal hilum

13 肝门静脉右后下支 right posteroinferior branch of hepatic portal vein

14 肝裸区 bare area of liver

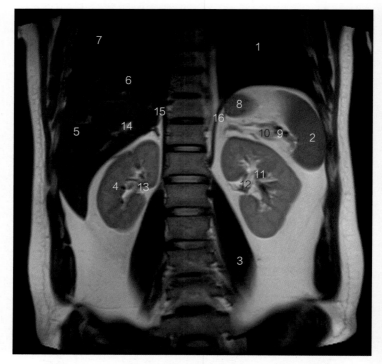

图 6-14　经左、右肾门后份的冠状断层 MR T₂加权图像

1　左肺下叶 inferior lobe of left lung

2　脾 spleen

3　腰大肌 psoas major

4　右肾 right kidney

5　肝右后叶 right posterior lobe of liver

6　肝裸区 bare area of liver

7　右肺下叶 inferior lobe of right lung

8　胃底 fundus of stomach

9　脾门 splenic hilum

10　胰尾 tail of pancreas

11　左肾 left kidney

12　左肾门 left renal hilum

13　右肾门 right renal hilum

14　肝门静脉右后下支 right posteroinferior branch of hepatic portal vein

15　右膈脚 right crus of diaphragm

16　左膈脚 left crus of diaphragm

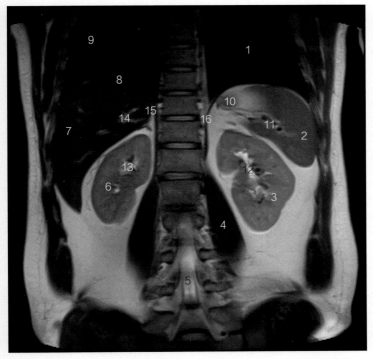

图 6-15 经左、右肾窦后份和脾门的冠状断层 MR T₂ 加权图像

1 左肺下叶 inferior lobe of left lung　　2 脾 spleen

3 左肾 left kidney　　4 腰大肌 psoas major

5 马尾 cauda equina　　6 右肾 right kidney

7 肝右后叶 right posterior lobe of liver　　8 肝裸区 bare area of liver

9 右肺下叶 inferior lobe of right lung　　10 胃底 fundus of stomach

11 脾门 splenic hilum　　12 左肾窦 left renal sinus

13 右肾窦 right renal sinus

14 肝门静脉右后下支 right posteroinferior branch of hepatic portal vein

15 右膈脚 right crus of diaphragm　　16 左膈脚 left crus of diaphragm

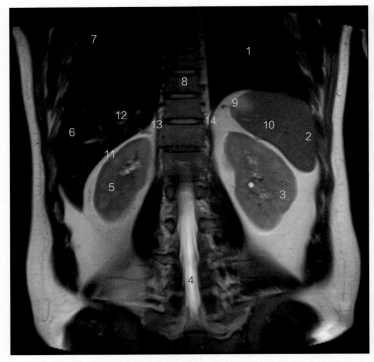

图 6-16　经马尾的冠状断层 MR T₂ 加权图像

1　左肺下叶 inferior lobe of left lung　　　2　脾 spleen

3　左肾 left kidney　　　4　马尾 cauda equina

5　右肾 right kidney

6　肝右后叶 right posterior lobe of liver

7　右肺下叶 inferior lobe of right lung

8　第 10 胸椎椎体 body of 10th thoracic vertebrae

9　胃脾隐窝 gastrosplenic recess　　　10　脾门 splenic hilum

11　右肝下间隙 right subhepatic space

12　肝门静脉右后下支 right posteroinferior branch of hepatic portal vein

13　右膈脚 right crus of diaphragm　　　14　左膈脚 left crus of diaphragm

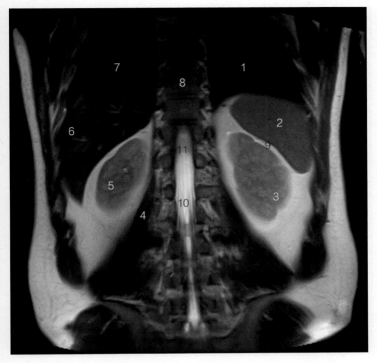

图 6-17 经脊髓圆锥和马尾的冠状断层 MR T₂ 加权图像

1　左肺下叶 inferior lobe of left lung　　　2　脾 spleen

3　左肾 left kidney　　　4　腰大肌 psoas major

5　右肾 right kidney　　　6　肝右后叶 right posterior lobe of liver

7　右肺下叶 inferior lobe of right lung

8　第 10 胸椎椎体 body of 10th thoracic vertebrae

9　脾肾隐窝 splenorenal recess　　　10　马尾 cauda equina

11　脊髓圆锥 conus medullaris

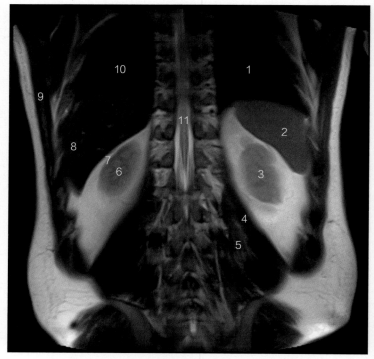

图 6-18　经脊髓的冠状断层 MR T₂加权图像

1	左肺下叶 inferior lobe of left lung	2	脾 spleen
3	左肾 left kidney	4	腰大肌 psoas major
5	竖脊肌 erector spinae	6	右肾 right kidney
7	右肝下间隙 right subhepatic space		
8	肝右后叶 right posterior lobe of liver	9	背阔肌 latissimus dorsi
10	右肺下叶 inferior lobe of right lung	11	脊髓 spinal cord

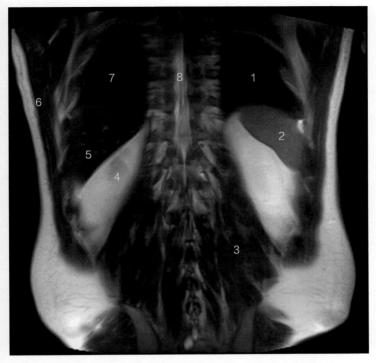

图 6-19 经右肾后极的冠状断层 MR T₂ 加权图像

1 左肺下叶 inferior lobe of left lung	2 脾 spleen
3 竖脊肌 erector spinae	
4 右肾后极 posterior pole of right kidney	
5 肝右后叶 right posterior lobe of liver	6 背阔肌 latissimus dorsi
7 右肺下叶 inferior lobe of right lung	8 脊髓 spinal cord

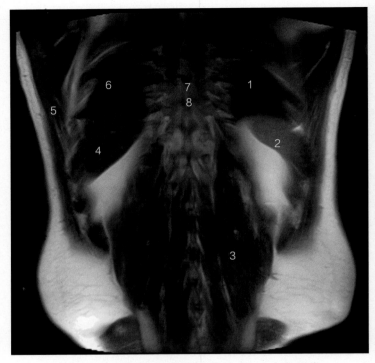

图 6-20 经椎管后壁的冠状断层 MR T₂ 加权图像

1 左肺下叶 inferior lobe of left lung	2 脾 spleen
3 竖脊肌 erector spinae	
4 肝右后叶 right posterior lobe of liver	5 背阔肌 latissimus dorsi
6 右肺下叶 inferior lobe of right lung	7 棘突 spinous process
8 椎管后壁 posterior wall of spinal canal	

第七章　腹部 B 超图像

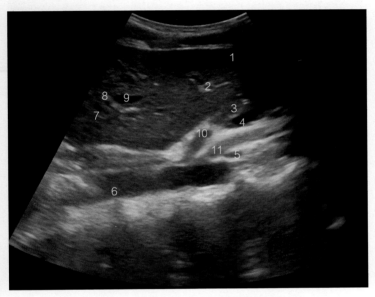

图 7-1　经腹主动脉肝左叶矢状切面图

1　肝左外叶下段　inferior segment of left lateral lobe of liver

2　肝门静脉左外下支　left lateroinferior branch of hepatic portal vein

3　胰 pancreas　　　　　　　　4　脾静脉 splenic vein

5　左肾静脉 left renal vein　　　　6　腹主动脉 abdominal aorta

7　肝左外叶上段 superior segment of left lateral lobe of liver

8　肝门静脉左外上支 left laterosuperior branch of hepatic portal vein

9　肝左静脉 left hepatic vein　　　10　腹腔干 celiac trunk

11　肠系膜上动脉 superior mesenteric artery

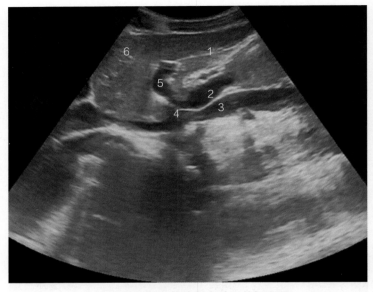

图 7-2 经下腔静脉肝左叶矢状切面图

1 肝圆韧带 ligamentum teres hepatis　　2 肝门静脉 hepatic portal vein

3 下腔静脉 inferior vena cava　　　　　4 肝尾状叶 caudate lobe of liver

5 肝门静脉左支矢状部 sagittal part of hepatic portal vein

6 肝左内叶 left medial lobe of liver

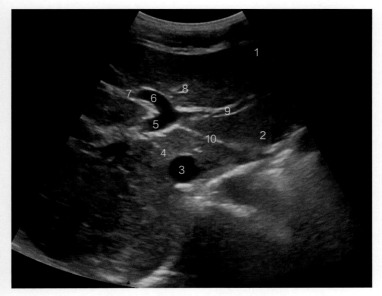

图 7-3　经剑突下肝左叶斜切面图

1　肝左外叶下段 inferior segment of left lateral lobe of liver

2　肝左外叶上段　superior segment of left lateral lobe of liver

3　下腔静脉 inferior vena cava

4　肝尾状叶 caudate lobe of liver

5　肝门静脉左支横部 transverse part of hepatic portal vein

6　肝门静脉左支矢状部　sagittal part of hepatic portal vein

7　肝门静脉左内叶支 left medial branch of hepatic portal vein

8　肝门静脉左外下支　left lateroinferior branch of hepatic portal vein

9　肝门静脉左外上支　left laterosuperior branch of hepatic portal vein

10　静脉韧带 ligamentum venosum

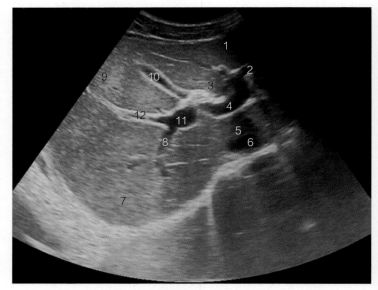

图 7-4　经第一肝门右肋下斜切面图

1　肝左外叶下段 inferior segment of left lateral lobe of liver

2　肝门静脉左外下支 left lateroinferior branch of hepatic portal vein

3　肝左内叶 left medial lobe of liver

4　肝门静脉左支横部 transverse part of hepatic portal vein

5　肝尾状叶 caudate lobe of liver

6　下腔静脉 inferior vena cava

7　肝右后叶 right posterior lobe of liver

8　肝门静脉右后支 posterior branch of right hepatic portal vein

9　肝右前叶 right anterior lobe of liver

10　胆囊 gallbladder

11　肝门静脉右支 right hepatic portal vein

12　肝门静脉右前支 anterior branch of right hepatic portal vein

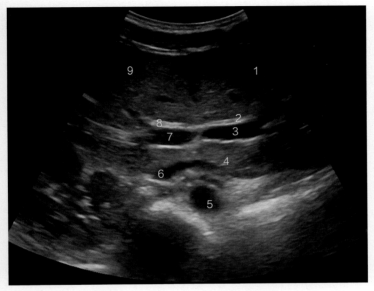

图 7-5 经第一肝门肋下斜切面图

1	肝左叶 left lobe of liver	2	肝左管 left hepatic duct

1　肝左叶 left lobe of liver　　　　　　　2　肝左管 left hepatic duct

3　肝门静脉左支横部 transverse part of left hepatic portal vein

4　肝尾状叶 caudate lobe of liver　　　　5　腹主动脉 abdominal aorta

6　下腔静脉 inferior vena cava

7　肝门静脉右支 right hepatic portal vein

8　肝右管 right hepatic duct　　　　　　9　肝右叶 right lobe of liver

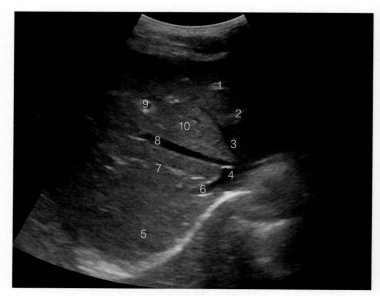

图 7-6　经第二肝门斜断面图

1　肝门静脉左外下支 left lateroinferior branch of hepatic portal vein

2　肝左外叶 left lateral lobe of liver　　3　肝左静脉 left hepatic vein

4　下腔静脉 inferior vena cava

5　肝右后叶 right posterior lobe of liver　6　肝右静脉 right hepatic vein

7　肝右前叶 right anterior lobe of liver　8　肝中静脉 middle hepatic vein

9　肝门静脉左支 left hepatic portal vein　10　肝左内叶 left medial lobe of liver

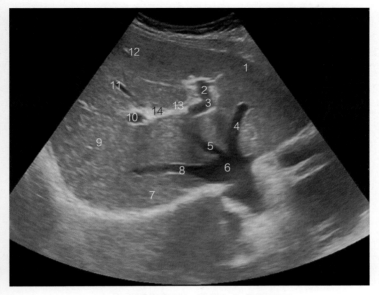

图 7-7　经剑突下经第二肝门斜断面图

1　肝左外叶 left lateral lobe of liver

2　肝门静脉左支矢状部 sagittal part of hepatic portal vein

3　肝门静脉左支角部 angular part of hepatic portal vein

4　肝左静脉 left hepatic vein　　　5　肝中静脉 middle hepatic vein

6　下腔静脉 inferior vena cava

7　肝右后叶 right posterior lobe of liver　　8　肝右静脉 right hepatic vein

9　肝右前叶 right anterior lobe of liver

10　肝门静脉右支 right hepatic portal vein

11　胆囊 gallbladder　　　　　12　肝左内叶 left medial lobe of liver

13　肝左管 left hepatic duct　　　14　肝右管 right hepatic duct

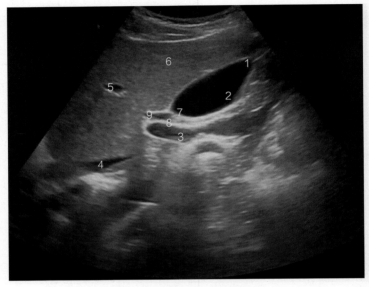

图 7-8　经肝 – 胆囊纵断面图

1　胆囊底 fundus of gallbladder　　　　2　胆囊体 body of gallbladder

3　肝门静脉右支　right hepatic portal vein

4　下腔静脉 inferior vena cava

5　肝门静脉右前支　anterior branch of right hepatic portal vein

6　肝右前叶　right anterior lobe of liver　　7　胆囊颈 neck of gallbladder

8　肝动脉 hepatic artery　　　　　　　　9　肝总管 common hepatic duct

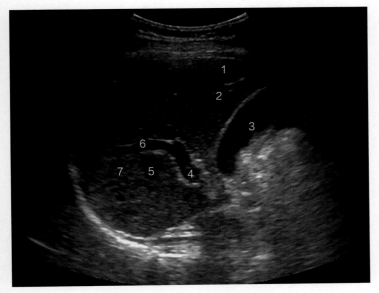

图 7-9　经肝右叶肋间斜切面图

1　肝右前叶 right anterior lobe of liver

2　肝门静脉右前支 anterior branch of right hepatic portal vein

3　胆囊 gallbladder　　　　　　4　肝门静脉右支 right hepatic portal vein

5　肝右静脉 right hepatic vein

6　肝门静脉右后支 posterior branch of right hepatic portal vein

7　肝右后叶　right posterior lobe of liver

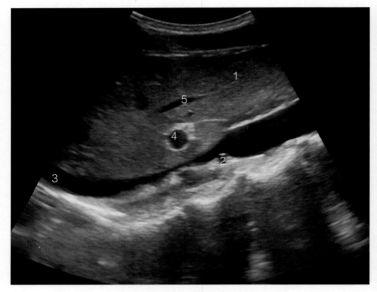

图 7-10 经下腔静脉肝右叶斜切面图

1 肝右叶 right lobe of liver
2 右肾动脉 right renal artery
3 下腔静脉 inferior vena cava
4 肝门静脉右支 right hepatic portal vein
5 肝右静脉 right hepatic vein

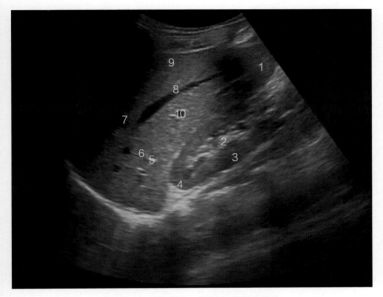

图 7-11　经肝 – 右肾矢状切面图

1　肝右后叶下段 inferior segment of right posterior lobe of liver

2　肾窦 renal sinus

3　肾实质 renal parenchyma

4　右肾上极 upper pole of right kidney

5　肝门静脉右后上支 right posterosuperior branch of hepatic portal vein

6　肝右后叶上段 superior segment of right posterior lobe of liver

7　肝右前叶上段 superior segment of right anterior lobe of liver

8　肝右静脉 right hepatic vein

9　肝右前叶下段 inferior segment of right anterior lobe of liver

10　肝门静脉右后下支 right posteroinferior branch of hepatic portal vein

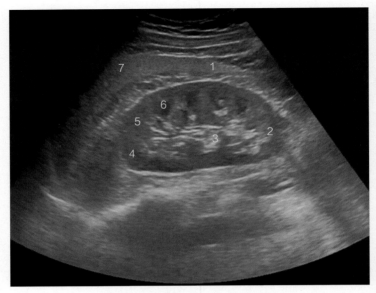

图 7-12　经脾 - 左肾矢状切面图

1　脾下极 lower pole of spleen　　　　2　左肾下极 lower pole of left kidney

3　肾窦 renal sinus　　　　　　　　　4　左肾上极 upper pole of left kidney

5　肾皮质 renal cortex　　　　　　　　6　肾锥体 renal pyramid

7　脾 spleen

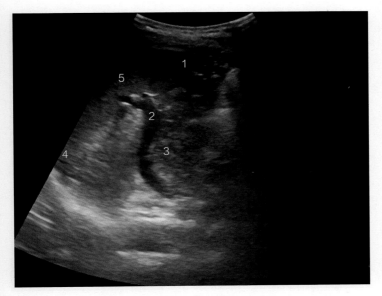

图 7-13　经脾－胰尾冠状切面图

1	脾下极 lower pole of spleen	2	脾静脉 splenic vein
3	胰尾 tail of pancreas	4	脾上极 upper pole of spleen
5	脾 spleen		

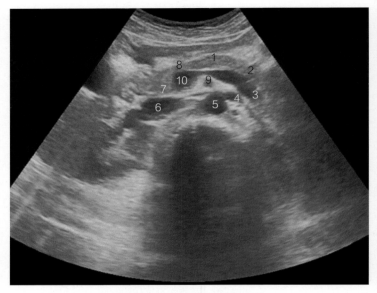

图 7-14 经胰腺长轴切面图

1 胰体 body of pancreas	2 胰尾 tail of pancreas
3 脾静脉 splenic vein	4 左肾静脉 left renal vein
5 腹主动脉 abdominal aorta	6 下腔静脉 inferior vena cava
7 胰头 head of pancreas	8 胰颈 neck of pancreas
9 肠系膜上动脉 superior mesenteric artery	
10 肠系膜上静脉 superior mesenteric vein	

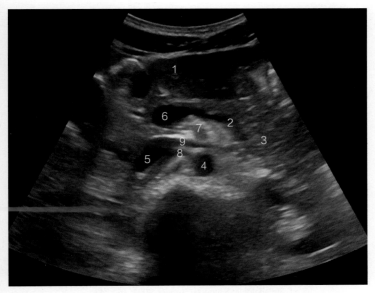

图 7-15　经肾血管平面的上腹部横切面图

1　肝左叶 left lobe of liver	2　脾静脉 splenic vein
3　胰尾 tail of pancreas	4　腹主动脉 abdominal aorta
5　下腔静脉 inferior vena cava	
6　肠系膜上静脉 superior mesenteric vein	
7　肠系膜上动脉 superior mesenteric artery	
8　右肾动脉 right renal artery	9　左肾静脉 left renal vein

推荐阅读文献

1. 刘树伟. 断层解剖学. 第 3 版. 北京：高等教育出版社，2017.
2. 刘树伟. 人体断层解剖学图谱. 济南：山东科学技术出版社，2011: 118-151.
3. 周进祝. 超声诊断学. 北京：人民卫生出版社，2011: 38-45.
4. 刘树伟，柳澄，胡三元. 腹部外科临床解剖学图谱. 济南：山东科学技术出版社，2006.
5. 刘树伟，邢子英. 腹部应用解剖学. 北京：高等教育出版社，2007.
6. 王振宇，徐文坚. 人体断面与影像解剖学. 第 3 版. 北京：人民卫生出版社，2010.
7. 徐峰. 人体断面解剖学图谱. 北京：人民卫生出版社，1989.
8. 张朝佑. 人体解剖学（上）. 第 3 版. 北京：人民卫生出版社，2009: 287-422, 589-607.
9. 赵振美，刘树伟，林祥涛，等. 右半肝内门静脉的断层影像解剖学研究. 解剖学报，2008, 39(5): 760-764.
10. 晋云，陈刚，张绍祥，等. 胰腺及其周围结构的多方位断层解剖研究. 第三军医大学学报，2007, 29(23): 2271-2273.
11. Bo WJ, Carr JJ, Krueger WA, et al. Basic Atlas of Sectional Anatomy with Correlated Imaging. 4th ed. Philadelphia: Saunders Elsevier, 2007: 160-243.
12. El-Khoury GY, Montgomery WJ, Bergman RA. Sectional Anatomy by MRI and CT. 3rd ed. Edinburgh：Churchill Livingstone, 2007.
13. Ellis H, Logan BM, Dixon AK. Human sectional anatomy. 3rd ed. London: hodder Arnold, 2007.
14. Heilmaier C, Sutter R, Lutz AM, et al. Mapping of hepatic vascular anatomy: dynamic contrastenhanced parallel MR imaging compared with 64-detector row CT. Radiology, 2007, 245(3): 872-880.
15. Federle MP, Rosado-de-Christenson ML, Woodward PJ, et al. Diagnostic and Surgical Imaging Anatomy: Chest, Abdomen, Pelvis. Salt Lske City: Amirsys Publishing, Inc., 2007.
16. Jinkins JR. Atlas of Neuroradiologic Embryology，Anatomy，and Variants. Philadelphia：Lippincott Williams & Wilkins，2000.
17. Laghi A. Multidector CT(64 Slices) of the liver: examination techniques. Eur Radiol, 2007, 17(3): 675-683.
18. Okahara M, Mori H, Kiyosue H, et al. Arterial supply to the pancreas; variations and cross-sectional anatomy. Abdom Imaging, 2010,35(2): 134-142.
19. Torigian DA, Hammell MK. Netter's Correlative Imaging Abdominal & Pelvic Anatomy. Philadelphia: Elsevier Saunders, 2013.